The Transparent Feather

With Blessings,
BJ Appelgren

The Transparent Feather

B J Appelgren

Zillah, Inc.
Charles Town, WV 25414

Zillah, Inc.
P.O.Box 887
Charles Town, WV 25414

Book and Cover Design: Bruce Appelgren
Front Cover Illustration: Molly Goldstein
Back Cover Photo: Tara Bell
www.transparentfeather.com

ISBN: 0-9619884-0-1
1. Personal growth, spirituality. 2. Death, dying. 3. Writing. 4. Morgan, Berry.

*To Berry Morgan, who believed for me,
and to the Otherworld, which comes to each of us
in its own way*

Imagination

The Celtic otherworld was and is accessible through that burning glass of the soul, the imagination. The original sense of the word 'imagination' has become warped into meaning 'a faculty to dream up illusory things'. But the imagination is nothing less than our doorway to the otherworld, it is the prime faculty of shamanic consciousness through which come the dreams, visions and ideas which we in turn implement in ordinary reality. We have to learn to trust the information that our meditations give us, trusting our imagination and our dreams, and sifting the answers the otherworld gives us.

- CAITLIN AND JOHN MATTHEWS, ENCYCLOPEDIA OF CELTIC WISDOM

Foreword

There are two worlds. One is the world of facts,
and the other is the world of possibilities.
In the world of facts, there are no possibilities;
in the world of possibilities, there are no facts.
-JG BENNETT

Berry Morgan had been a fiction writer for *The New Yorker* magazine from 1966 to 1988, receiving two Houghton Mifflin Literary Fellowship awards for her novel *Pursuit* in 1966 and what had originated as a collection of short stories, *The Mystic Adventures of Roxie Stoner*, in 1974. She was originally from Port Gibson, Mississippi, later moving with her children to West Virginia.

The Transparent Feather is about the year-and-a-half I spent visiting with Berry at the end of her life. When I first met her, I still had trouble recognizing my guiding inner voice, let alone hearing it and following its counsel. Something about the mix of our personalities, however, finally changed that for me.

Prologue—Finding A Feather

What we see depends mainly on what we look for.
-SIR JOHN LUBBOCK

As I neared the end of our neighborhood business district, I slowed my pace, luxuriating in the increasing sunlight of a late winter day that promised spring.

Almost sixty years old, living in this West Virginia town for over twenty years and still feeling like a newcomer. Is this how it is to be an adult? Nothing ever feels as familiar as the environment of childhood. Or had my childhood's demand for vigilance distorted my perception?

Not sure of what I was seeing, I bent over to pick up what turned out to be a gossamer feather. It was about four inches long and rather wide, brown-and-white striped. Yet, when held up, I could see right through it. Marvelling over its enigmatic transparency, I felt that within me a lens had focused.

This feather so moved me, even though it was barely present. Isn't life like that? Material, yet never far from being seen through—to what? More life, but in greater depth? Subtlety? Complexity? When I concentrated on the feather, it took on weight and presence. All its details clarified. Yet if I fixed my gaze there, I'd never see all that lies beyond it.

I took the feather home and stuck it among the crystals of a rock that sat atop my desktop computer. Every now and then, taking a thoughtful break from writing, I would hold the feather in my hand, stroking it, alternately looking at it and then, without losing awareness of its presence, look through it.

One day, in a hurry to run some errands, I noticed an amazingly similar feather in our driveway. Picking it up gingerly because it looked dirty, maybe just broken leaves stuck to its down, I considered saving it. Oh, I have one so much like it—even dirt on its down when I'd first found it—and, besides, I was in a hurry. I poked it into the nearby ground cover with the idea of coming back for it and promptly forgot all about it.

9

Almost a week later, when my friend Tara and I were sitting in front of the computer, she excitedly told me about a feather she'd found and an interesting book about feathers.

"Hey, I have an incredible feather!" I said, interrupting her and reaching up to get it. But it wasn't there. My heart sank. Had the gossamer feather in the driveway fallen down from the crystal and stuck to my clothing? Maybe when it had drifted to the ground near the car, I noticed it. Given a chance to reclaim it, I'd been in too much of a hurry. Now it was gone.

After Tara left, feeling vaguely ashamed of my attachment, I strode out to the driveway and crouched down to search the nearby ground cover, raking it with my fingers, hoping to come up with something. How could I find it in such a tangle of vines or had the wind carried it away?

No sign of the feather. Yet, hadn't it already done its work? I carried it in my heart, a signpost pointing to a different reality—it drove me to embark on this book. Actually, there were two catalysts...the feather and, of course, Berry.

For almost the year-and-a-half Berry lived in a nearby nursing home, I visited her three times a week. She had wanted to give her family some casual memoirs and was no longer able to hold a pen. Initially, she refused my offers to take dictation. However, after I told her of my dissatisfaction with some stories I'd written about mysterious events in my life, she suggested an exchange. She, who had been published by *The New Yorker* and Houghton Mifflin years before, would work with me on improving my writing!

Over the time of our friendship, Berry's spiritual embrace slowly confirmed in me a new outlook. Her acknowledgment helped me accept the ethereal events that had demonstrated repeatedly the existence of a loving, mysterious universe.

As Berry and I looked back upon our lives, as she listened without cynicism, my wish grew to fully embrace the strange happenings I had been driven to share with her. I've come to learn it wasn't their nature to be so elusive; it was something I had been doing that made them seem so. After Berry's death, my yearning for greater understanding increased. Writing about our time together has lengthened our unique collaboration. Because of Berry, I have been attending ever more closely to the reality seen beyond the feather.

Mary Jane's Introduction

For all prayer is answered. Don't tell God how to answer it.
- EDGAR CAYCE READING 4028-1

It wasn't until I'd already known Berry for some time that I recalled an almost negligible moment that happened perhaps as long as a year before I met her.

On the way to do some errands in my car, I am lamenting that at 58 years old, I still lack direction in life. As I am about to turn the first corner away from home, my eyes glance across the T of the road to the rows of gravestones in the cemetery. I wish I had a mentor, I say to myself. Surely, there's some old lady living around here I could really talk with about life.

I had long forgotten that quickly-made wish when Mary Jane first introduced me to Berry. At the time, I was working for the Federal Emergency Management Agency (FEMA). They had needed 200 human service operators to take applications for aid over the telephone. As emergency personnel, our hours changed often and the threat of being laid off hung over us, adding to the atmosphere of anxiety inherent in speaking with so many individuals who had recently experienced disaster.

Here I was, at an age when most people were retiring, going to fortieth class reunions, and smiling at grandchildren they could enjoy in ways they could not enjoy their own children. Instead, I was feeling I might finally be coming of age. I had always thought I was going to be a late bloomer. At thirty-nine, I was just earning a degree in social work and getting married. Nevertheless, I had to wait still another generation before feeling on the verge of being connected to a larger sense of purpose.

Not that I knew yet how it was going to manifest; it was my relationship with Berry that made me think it could. But I'm getting ahead of myself. I had just met Berry in February. Mary Jane, a mutual friend, introduced us. She was a perky blue-eyed nurse, her youthful beauty contradicting years of experience working with hospice. I had phoned her for a Therapeutic Touch appointment to relax me, to help me cope with driving to FEMA on the icy mountain road.

"Why don't I give you a treatment at your home?" Mary Jane asked. "I'm going through Charles Town anyway, visiting a family friend in a nursing home. She used to be a writer, had some stories published in *The New Yorker*." Then, as if just remembering, she added, "Actually, she's quite a character. I think you'd like her. Why don't you come with me?" She laughed, saying, "Last time I was there she told me she was getting ready to shed her body and grow into her spiritual life."

Glad to be in Mary Jane's bright aura of optimism, I agreed to go, though I've always disliked nursing homes. Both of my mother's parents had lived in them for years. I remembered dark rooms with no beauty or privacy, an unpleasant stench, and people who talked condescendingly. My grandmother had been addicted to painkillers for 11 years, refusing rehab for a broken hip. Had depression made her choose to die that way?

Self-conscious about being there, I felt a bit intrusive. This was Berry's home now and we hadn't even asked her permission for me to visit. I stood there trying to be inconspicuous while observing the sterile environment—no rugs or curtains, floors painfully shiny from too many chemicals, the monotonous prattle of television in the background, clattering that echoed through the halls, the sounds layered by a counterpoint of voices calling out for help. I made myself ignore them.

Berry's hospital bed lay parallel the picture window on her left. Open blinds revealed the ubiquitous bird feeder and a wide lawn appearing to stretch right up to the Blue Ridge Mountains. A few plants and an elderly bouquet were on the window sill, TV enthroned high on the wall opposite the foot of her bed.

Berry invited me to sit to her right while Mary Jane chirped greetings, dragging a chair for herself to the space between the bed and window. Berry looked emaciated and frail, her long bones everywhere apparent under translucent skin, straight gray hair cut short without style, combed straight back from her face. Yet her engaging dark eyes were intelligent and lively.

Mary Jane introduced us as I was getting seated. Then, after sitting down herself, she said to Berry, "How do you feel about being in the nursing home?" I hadn't been prepared for her directness, but figured she was using her experience as a hospice nurse to encourage Berry to air her feelings. Mary Jane had told me on the way over that Berry would never complain to her daughter, who wept over having to bring her mother there.

Berry answered casually, "I don't mind. I could understand the need. Slowly, she said, as if considering various possibilities, "I don't really know what this place is." Did she mean she didn't know where she was? Then she added, "...a kind of holding pen, I suppose." I laughed at her unexpected frankness. Mary Jane didn't. Had I made a social blunder? Berry turned her face to me and flashed a shrewd smile—we understood each other.

Mary Jane pulled a voice-activated tape recorder out of her purse. Berry had told her she wanted to write memoirs to leave to her family but she was already unable to write by hand anymore. Mary Jane's operating instructions didn't get very far. The technology seemed to stymie Berry, or maybe, she just wasn't interested. Either way, she couldn't hear her own voice, the sound reedy and weak. Her hands shook intensely, fingers seeming too feeble and, finally, even with glasses, she couldn't make out the tiny labels on the buttons. However, the scene started me thinking—it might be fun taking dictation from a published writer.

Uncertain Beginning

*The future enters into us, in order to transform itself in us,
long before it happens.*
- RAINER MARIA RILKE

My shift at FEMA, from 10:00 a.m. to 4:00 p.m., would allow me
to visit Berry first thing in the morning if I chose to call on her
again. Doubtful whether I wanted to be going there, my internal
dialogue would ask, If I start visiting, won't she begin expecting
me? Would I be able to keep it up, adding these visits to my To-Do
List? I was already feeling like I didn't have enough time to complete yet another of my latest projects, readying the layout for the
Healing Arts Directory, a guide to local alternative and complementary health practitioners.

After several days of returning to the idea of visiting Berry
again, I simply got myself out of the house early one morning,
drove up to the tidy looking nursing home, and signed the guest
register in the foyer. The book shared a small faux baroque table
with a clock—roman numerals and flowers on its face—and a vase
holding an artificial bouquet. It was almost eight o'clock. The air
of the foyer smelled mustier than inside the building itself.
According to the register, I was the first visitor of the day.

The location of Berry's room required I walk almost the full
length of the building. Staff was nowhere in sight. Making their
rounds, I supposed. From her doorway, I could see Berry lying on
her side, propped up on her right elbow, looking very uncomfortable, her shoulders contracted close to her head. I entered just as
she was about to poke at her breakfast. She noticed me and waved
me closer.

"Oh, hello! Sit down, Dear. Move the basket. You can put it
over here against the railing," she said, pointing behind her. The
burgeoning basket had a rosary of glittering black beads hanging
from the handle. It held a notebook, pen, eye glasses, Advil, and
napkins.

I apologized, "I'm sorry for coming so early in the day."

"You can't come too early. I've been up for hours. I wake up around four and can't get back to sleep. Pull the curtain, won't you?" From against the wall, I slid the curtain out that gave her some privacy from her roommate. Then, in a stage whisper she added, "That old bag is always trying to eavesdrop. And she has nothing nice to say about anything." I chuckled nervously wondering if Berry was intending to be funny.

Conversation was a bit stilted at first. She asked where I came from. "Chicago," I said. Then she told me she was born in Port Gibson, Mississippi. I heard it as Fort Gibson and we took some time to straighten that out.

"Berry is a family name," she revealed. "My real name is Betty." Even though I'd only recently met her, I couldn't imagine her with that apple-pie identity. Her grandparents, her mother's parents, she said, were a large part of her early childhood. "We lived with them. My grandfather was a banker, my grandmother the heart of the household. She was the one who introduced us all to literature." Berry's face lightened for a moment as she looked at a vision with her inner eye. "I thought my mother was someone quite grand, like a movie star, very beautiful and intelligent."

After Berry learned I was married but had no children, she asked about my childhood family. Maybe it was her planned memoir that brought up so much thought of childhood. Yet right from the beginning, her candor made me feel I could say anything to her.

Within a couple of weeks of visiting regularly, our chats acquired an easy familiarity. Perhaps not knowing Berry in life outside the nursing home provided a feeling of safety, like when you talk to a stranger on a long-distance bus trip. Or maybe knowing Berry was soon supposed to die created an abnormal sense of shared privacy. Whatever the cause, we were never at a loss for topics of conversation.

"Is your mother still alive?" she asked.

"No," I said, "she died in '91."

"What was she like?"

I couldn't remember anyone ever asking about her that way. A strange thought crossed my mind, that Berry was checking to see if Mom would make a good character in a book.

"She was very beautiful when she was younger. You should see my parents' wedding picture."

"Would you bring it?" Berry asked

I nodded, saying, "They looked like movie stars, too. In fact, they said the photographer later became famous photographing the stars in Hollywood. My mother always seemed dissatisfied with life. Aside from spending time with old friends, she was relentless about shopping—not for big or expensive things, just a steady stream of ..." I groped for words "...consolation prizes."

Berry chuckled and I continued. "To her friends, she seemed to have a very gentle manner but at home her anger slipped out in stinging barbs."

"Ah, your mom played to an audience." Berry summarized.

I laughed at her quick appraisal. "My mom never said anything positive to us kids unless one of her friends did, expecting her to agree. But you got the feeling she really hadn't noticed whatever it was until someone else pointed it out, it having no value to her until then."

"My mother was just the opposite," Berry said. "She was very independent and, likewise, seemed to think we could do anything. She entered a poem of mine in a contest and we won two hundred dollars—an enormous amount of money at that time which she used toward purchasing a car. However, I remember taking care of her from early on, then working at a job for pay from the age of fifteen. My mother had become very sick in her late twenties, the same unidentified illness I have, though my symptoms didn't show up until a lot later."

Berry appeared to have something like Parkinson's Disease. Her hands shook violently and her mind was clear. She was completely bedridden, fearful of breaking a bone, and complaining of severe pain when they tried to give her physical therapy.

She said, "I started taking care of my mother when I was only seven. At that time, we went to Colorado by train, leaving my little brother in the care of my grandparents. Still, Mother didn't die until she was 76, living with my family in New Orleans right to the end. She had become quite paranoid by that time, though, always telling people stories about how badly we were treating her. I would get peculiarly probing phone calls from suspicious friends and relatives, checking up on us to make sure we hadn't done her in."

I imagined how awful it would be to have to defend yourself from a person you were caring for. But, then, remembering how withdrawn and angry I had become as a child, I wondered if my parents hadn't felt that way about me.

I admitted to Berry that throughout my life my mother told everyone what a difficult baby I had been. Actually, her words were, what a *bad* baby I had been. As an infant I cried inconsolably. Maybe to protect me from her frustration, the doctor told her to just let me cry myself to exhaustion. It wasn't until I was an adult that I heard about babies suffering from colic. It surprised me to hear those mothers sounding so sympathetic toward their children. On the other hand, Mom always raved about what an easy child my older brother Jerry had been. She could just stick him in the corner with a toy and leave him there for hours. He'd never bother her like I did.

"By the time I was an adult," I said, "I learned that, if I behaved like the mother, my mom and I could get along, but I never could depend on her to be the mother if I needed emotional support."

I wanted Berry to know that the relationship between Mom and I did improve. "We talked on the phone regularly and I visited her in Chicago every year. Near the end of her life after she had been diagnosed with colon cancer, she really went through a transformation."

Mothers' Love

The subject tonight is Love
And for tomorrow night as well.
As a matter of fact I know of no better topic
For us to discuss
Until we all
Die!

- HAFIZ, TRANSLATED BY DANIEL LADINSKY

"At the time of her first surgery," I said, "Mom would, for the first time in my life, sometimes say 'I love you' when we were saying good-bye on the phone."

Berry seemed surprised, almost relieved—as if saying 'I love you' to her children was something she had been able to do.

Then I told Berry how after Mom was diagnosed a couple of years later with a return of the cancer and that it was inoperable, she became even more demonstrative. I had been living out here for years by then and had to schedule time off from work to visit and help make arrangements for her care in Chicago. My ex-sister-in-law had already connected her with hospice. They had a nurse, a homemaker, and an aide come out a total of five times during the week. By the end of my visit we found her a live-in caregiver.

"Mom was so grateful for everyone's help, she was saying 'I love you' to everyone. I got high from her exuding so much love. It also made me sad to see how much nurturing she had missed out on all her life because she had never been able to say it before."

Berry looked into my eyes with interest and sympathy.

"One day, as I was assisting Mom with her daily bath, she said to me, 'I love you for who you are.' It caught my breath. I'd waited all my life to hear that from her. Of course, she'd waited all her life to be able to say it." It didn't seem strange to be telling all this to Berry.

"There was a time in the past I'd felt so bitter toward Mom that I wondered what I would do when she was dying. I imagined using this vulnerable time to get back at her by throwing her emotional neglect in her face, explaining my lifelong struggle against feeling suicidal and ill. 'You love me for who I am?' I imagined asking. 'Since when? All you ever did was correct me and make fun of my childhood needs. Can you even begin to imagine how I longed for your approval? To Jerry and me, there was never a spontaneous hug, or a show of pride in anything we did.

"Instead, I found myself being tender, wanting her to have a good death, listening to her take stock of her life."

When I finished what I'd been saying, Berry and I just looked at each other for awhile, okay with silence. Sitting like that allowed me to return from what felt like a visit to Mom's condo ten years before.

Berry said she had been her mother's first child and at an early age had been drafted to provide care for her. "One of the tasks I was given was to read aloud to her. I read the newspaper and all the classics and we would discuss everything! I've come to realize it was quite an education."

Even seated, I was looking down at Berry, watching her face soften as I said, "I can't imagine what it would have been like to spend that amount of time conversing with my mom about the meaning of anything. We never had discussions in our house—and they didn't read to us, either."

She thought about that. Then, she returned to her description. "I took care of my little brother, too. I loved him dearly. I thought he was so handsome with his red hair. Glad to have his company, I guess, though he made it clear I was overbearing—maybe it was like having two mothers. Do you have any siblings besides your brother?"

"No, just him."

"Does he live around here? Is he married?"

"He still lives near Chicago—with his wife Linda. He has three grown daughters from his first marriage. One lives with her mother. The others live in Boulder and Austin."

"You mentioned he was older, right?"

"By five years."

Berry said, "That's a big age difference to kids. Were you close?"

"No, though we're friends now. I think he felt as neglected by our parents as I did, but when he saw me, the new baby, getting the attention any newborn needs, he seemed to take out his anger on me and I rarely felt protected. Only when the noise of our fighting annoyed our parents would they intervene. They were of the persuasion that the children have to learn to work it out for themselves. We don't have a lot of interests in common though Jerry now seems to admire my intellect. I think he's been impressed and a little mystified by my interests. They're so different from his. He was really into cars and now computers. I always admired his patience, teaching himself how to weld and re-configure his car from reading books.

"I think he feels guilty about how he treated me when we were kids. Maybe he should, but not for the reason he thinks. I doubt he remembers teasing me about my looks and scaring me on a daily basis. After all, he was a child himself. Just last year he told me he wondered if my emotional difficulties growing up were from his having dropped me on my head as a baby. As soon as he said it, I remembered the terrible jolt. And I recalled how I would never let anyone pick me up throughout my childhood. I'd always wondered why I was so fearful of that when other kids seemed to love it."

Berry looked at me with curiosity, nodding and waiting for me to continue. I told her how my uncles would give the cousins highly coveted rides up on their shoulders or spin them around by their hands.

"The threat of that little game would send me into hiding. But the most difficult part of childhood, was feeling so blue. It followed the same pattern well into my twenties. I'd be depressed for a long period of time and suddenly become what, by contrast, seemed high—a day or two of contentment and hope. Yet, I came to dread even that short-lived feeling of well-being because I understood it was also the precursor to another plummet."

"What changed that?"

I recalled how changing my diet helped, but first, I went for therapy in college and found it unexpectedly helpful. Just the emotional intimacy of talking with someone who wasn't judgmental was healing in itself. After college, a friend lent me a book by Carl G. Jung—*Modern Man in Search of His Soul.* Coincidently, another friend gave me *Man and His Symbols,* written by Jung and several of his students. When I read Jung's autobiography—*Memories, Dreams, Reflections*—I thought how great it would be, as an artist, to have therapy with someone who understood visual language and who connected it with spiritual experience. So I wrote to the Jung Institute in Switzerland and they gave me the name of a woman who, at that time, was the only Jungian analyst in Chicago.

"There was only one Jungian?" Berry asked.

"It's hard to believe, isn't it? But, if you think about his training students that came from all over the world, I was lucky to find one just a couple of miles from where I was living. Her name was June Singer and she became very well known, wrote a few books."

"Oh, I heard of her," Berry said, naming one of the books, *Boundaries of the Soul.*

Nodding, I said, "You know how Jungians put a lot of stock in the dream a patient brings to their first session. It's supposed to be a pretty good indicator of how therapy might progress or whether the patient is ready for change. Well, the night before seeing her the first time, I dreamed she held me in her lap like a toddler. In therapy, it was such a relief to show her my art work without having to twist it into words." I felt tension melt away from my body as I spoke.

Conditions

You already have the precious mixture
that will make you well. Use it.
-Rumi

"Where did you study art?" Berry asked.

"The Art Institute of Chicago."

Berry smiled. "My mother studied there." Then with a look of disappointment added, "But she never finished her degree. It was hard on a woman to be in the city on her own at that time."

Had her mother regretted not staying? I wondered, but didn't ask. Instead, I projected my own scenario, "It can be pretty scary there. Every day there was murder in the headlines and, taking the el downtown, I was regularly accosted. Not really dangerous stuff, just creepy. Men leaned on you when they stood next to you or put a hand on your knee and then ran out the door at a station."

We laughed at the foolishness of it.

Berry and I talked about family many times. During another visit, she claimed she'd never struggled with depression yet she insisted, "In order to be creative, I always needed to drink. I could do nothing without alcohol."

I asked, "Do you think you would have needed to drink if you could have thought of yourself as depressed?" She laughed at first but then you could see her take the words in, though we talked no more about it.

Another time Berry confided, "I was a terrible mother. I would drink throughout the night, my manuscript spread out on the basement floor. Drinking and making revisions. I don't know who was taking care of the kids. People were always angry with me for drinking. I didn't care. I had to write."

I almost wished I could feel so driven. In my life, there were always so many projects. I'd go from one to another, my interests in a constant state of flux, never staying with anything long enough to really develop it. A teacher of mine once reprimanded me, 'You act as though you have all the time in the world.' But what was I supposed to be doing?

Pointing to the wardrobe in the corner, Berry said, "I keep sherry in the closet. They let me have a half cup in the evening." I hoped she wasn't going to have me fetch it. Instead, she asked, "Don't *you* ever drink?"

"I can't anymore. The smallest amount of alcohol hurts my guts so badly. It's probably a good thing I have such an extreme reaction. I'd likely be alcoholic if I could tolerate it. Liqueurs would be my poison of choice: Kalua or fruit brandy, Bailey's Irish creme, Creme de Cacao—each mixed with cream so there'd be plenty of fat, too. Hmmmm, my mouth is watering just thinking of it," I admitted.

We grinned at each other. "Also," I added, "alcohol aggravates celiac disease. Celiac is probably why I cried so much when I was a baby. And why I was so depressed."

Most people don't know about celiac disease—intolerance to the gluten protein found in most grains—but Berry surprised me by saying, "I have a friend who almost died from it. She was just wasting away—and with three young children. The doctors couldn't figure out what was wrong."

"What happened to her?" I asked.

"Someone finally thought of testing her for celiac disease. They put her on a special diet. It was miraculous. She made a complete recovery after being so near death."

Warming to my favorite topic of drug-free health care, I launched into a lecture.

"It's one of the few life-threatening conditions the medical profession is willing to concede can be controlled completely by diet. I think it hadn't been until the nineteen-forties that the medical world really became more aware of it, although it had been identified fifty years before. Being unable to get flour during the war made them more cognizant. Sick babies became well. When they had been eating bread or crackers, they had been dying in spite of being well-fed. Doctors thought it was marasmus, you know, neglect, but these babies weren't being ignored in overcrowded

23

orphanages. The celia in the small intestine go flat from a reaction to gluten so the body simply can't absorb nutrients and the person essentially starves to death."

"Is that what happens?" Berry said, sounding genuinely interested. Her tone took me by surprise. I was more used to a covert annoyance, people wondering how they could be good hosts when I made it impossible for them to feed me. Berry asked, "How did you find out what was making you sick?"

"In college I finally made some progress in controlling symptoms by avoiding bread. I had been bloated all my life, but worse than that was suddenly getting the shakes, going noticeably pale, and breaking into a cold sweat. If I were outside, I'd have to sit wherever I was. Sometimes, it was so intense I'd burst into tears, unable to go on. I'd just sit down on the curb."

Berry was shaking her head or, rather, rolling it from side to side on the pillow.

"Learning to control it," I said, "was an accident, really. I'd been sick with mononucleosis and a friend had given me a book on nutrition. It said that some of the symptoms I was having might be caused by low blood sugar and it suggested ways to keep the level even, including eating only whole grains. At that time it was so hard to find whole grain bread that, when I couldn't, I just didn't eat any. When I didn't have bread, there were no attacks." After a pause, I added, "You know, my physical suffering may have been from celiac disease but it also seems too good a metaphor for the feeling of alienation I'd always had." Berry raised her eyebrows, waiting for me to finish the thought. "I couldn't stomach what for most people is the staff of life."

Taking Comfort

*There is no duty we so much underrate
as the duty of being happy. By being happy,
we sow enormous benefits upon the world.*
- Robert Louis Stevenson

Visiting Berry was providing a sort of comfort I hadn't ever expected to experience. It reminded me of what I'd heard people recount with nostalgic tenderness—the reassurance they got coming home from school to tell their moms about what happened that day.

I never had to explain to Berry why something caught my interest. I regaled her with stories about FEMA, disasters you never heard about in the newspaper, eccentricities of my co-workers, like the woman who angrily defied management's uncommon concern she might be overdoing it by refusing to take breaks, cutthroat competition among employees hoping for better jobs, the difficulties the contractor was having putting windows into a building which was once a bunker with three-foot thick walls, how the federal marshalls escorted away someone who was trying to hire a hit man over the Internet from a government work station. I also told her that since I had gotten my permanent ID, the guards didn't greet me in the morning in the old way any more. 'Good morning, Ma'am. Any cameras, guns, or explosives?' I missed the strange humor of it.

I had gone through a period of several weeks where I was feeling so tired at lunchtime, I would escape to my car to take a two-minute hypno-nap. "At least I'm using one skill from the hypnosis course I completed last December," I told Berry.

"How do you take a hypno-nap?"

"It's usually real easy. But you should have seen what happened last night. I had to go to a meeting with the Healing Arts Council—seven of us who voluntarily organize public events on alternative medicine.

"I was so sleepy driving to the restaurant to have dinner with them, I was practically dreaming about arriving early enough to

25

squeeze in a hypno-nap beforehand. In two minutes you can feel as well-rested as if you'd had a two-hour nap.... That's the suggestion I give to myself."

Berry lay back. "Would you crank up the bed some?" I went to the foot, crouching down to slowly turn the crank. She signalled me when to stop.

"Do you know Two Blocks West? I asked.

"No," she said, shaking her head.

I told her the whole story. It's kind of a classy restaurant in Winchester even though the entrance is in the alley across from the the back door of a popular shoe store. Low lighting, white table cloths, small vases of fresias, very elegant. Our gathering was a celebration and meeting to evaluate the most recent event we sponsored with James Gordon, an M.D. famous for his alternative approach to medicine.

I had stepped into the ladies' room before searching for our reserved table. A glance in the mirror caused me to groan aloud. I looked as tired as I felt, my face an unseemly shade of gray. I thought a hypno-nap would take just a few minutes. I could do it right there, but just as I sat down someone knocked on the door frantically. I called out and told them to wait a moment, but before ten seconds passed the person knocked again. Hadn't they heard me? Okay! Hang on. I just got here myself, I yelled. An apologetic but desperate woman answered, saying she was sorry. It was kind of an emergency.

So I scrubbed my idea, finished my legitimate business, and made way for the lady who gave me an embarrassed smile as we exchanged places in the narrow hallway. I caught sight of a small table half hidden by a large fern in the almost empty back room and figured maybe I could sit there quietly for a moment.

I described exactly what I did. "With my elbow on the table I put my hand to my forehead, closed my eyes, and took a deep breath. Ahhhhhh. Suddenly a voice hissed into my ear, 'Would you like a drink before dinner or are you waiting for someone?'"

"Oh, no," Berry said, rolling her eyes.

"I hadn't seen any waiter around before I sat down. Anyway,

I answered him stupidly, 'I'm with the Healing Arts Council.'"

"'Oh, their table is in the other room,' he proclaimed, waiting to escort me to my proper place. It really is easy to do a hypno-nap." I reiterated.

"Not in a public place, apparently," countered Berry.

"Well, at the appointed table, I was glad to see no one from our party had arrived yet. I thought I still had time to do it."

"You certainly can be focused when you want to be."

A sore point I ignored, but I finished explaining what had happened. I deflected further attention from the waiter by telling him that I would wait for the others before ordering. When I sat down again, I breathed deeply, cherishing the quiet. Elbow on the table once more, I resisted the temptation to just put my tired head down and go to sleep. I closed my eyes and began to count down from twenty. Nineteen. Eighteen. Seventeen. At sixteen. I felt a gentle touch on my left shoulder and looked up into Tom's smiling face. He's a retired medical doctor in our group, a handsome, balding man, always exuding a lot of energy and enthusiasm, which, at that moment, I was resenting.

There was only one thing to do. I asked him to please excuse me while I took a quick hypno-nap. I told him I could do it right there, that I just needed a couple of minutes of quiet to revive from my late afternoon slump.

Once again, with elbow on the table, I rested my forehead on my hand, closed my eyes, and counted back from twenty. I explained to Berry how I visualize each number being smoothly written, white on a black background. At zero I give myself the suggestion to feel really well-rested, as if having just taken a long nap, giving me all the energy I need for the rest of the evening, allowing me to fall asleep at home when it's time for bed.

I reinforce the suggestion and the ability to nap by adding, It's amazing how well-rested I can be by taking just a couple of minutes to nap in this way. And each time I practice, I can go deeper more quickly. Then, to bring me back to ordinary alertness, I count up to five saying, One, ready to return from the nap; two, physically relaxed and well-rested; three, mentally clear and alert;

four, enjoying one more second of this wonderful refreshing rest; and five, eyes wide open, wide awake and alert. Feeling great!

"Then," demonstrating to Berry, "I smile with absurd zeal to make myself laugh."

Berry laughed, too. She looked a little more rested herself.

"When I lifted my face, Dr. Tom, who had seated himself beside me, was looking straight into my eyes. He gasped, startling me.

"'What did you do?' he asked. 'Your face is all pink. How long will that last?' He was really excited. I explained the whole process to him. The wonderful thing is that the more you practice, the faster you can do it—usually," I added, thinking back to my stuttering start. "And it only took practicing once a day for a couple of weeks to learn."

Residence

*Practice SEEING heaven on earth
so you can CREATE heaven on earth.*
- Rob Brezsny, Free Will Astrology Newsletter

The visits were developing a familiar rhythm. Berry would invite me to sit, first having me close the privacy curtain, adjust the blinds, and then move the basket from the nicely padded guest chair to her bed. We'd adjust the bed if needed. Then she'd give me a quick synopsis of what had happened or who had visited as I settled in.

"I didn't get to sleep 'til late last night," she told me one day, pointing toward her roommate. Frowning and shaking her head, she added, "The shrew's relatives stayed until 10:00 p.m. Made plenty of noise, laughing and talking."

How could she stand the lack of privacy? I wouldn't say it, though, not wanting to feed any negative feelings. Wasn't life in a nursing home hard enough? Since she seemed to dislike her room-mate, I never conversed with the woman beyond an initial greet-ing. On another day, the roommate's daughter, son-in-law and grandchildren were there. I was reminded of how Berry had ardently described their husky size and the sweets they invariably brought, always offering to share them with her. If I were as upset with them as Berry had sounded, I would act distant and cool. Berry, on the other hand, was sweet as treacle to them. There was no way they'd ever suspect she didn't love their company. It made me wonder if she was fooling me, too.

Berry usually took the inevitable inconveniences of the nursing home in stride. She explained her state of acceptance. "Actually, I have nothing to do here. I can spend my time praying and think-ing, making my peace with the world. I'm ready to go."

She told me she had taught creative writing and American lit-erature at several colleges in Washington, D.C. while still farming outside of town. "I got the university jobs without having the usual credentials, just the fact of my writing and winning a Houghton Mifflin Literary Fellowship. I loved farming and need-ed to keep doing it to survive. The university staff were irked over my not having 'real' credentials."

Berry's farm was near the back road to Winchester. I told her about my having lived just up the way from her at Claymont for three-and-a-half years. She laughed, wondering how it was we'd never met. Claymont was an intentional community. I was one of about seventy people who'd come from all over to help establish it in 1974.

She told me, "I've had a few people from there live at my farm over the years. Do you know Georgia?"

"She's a friend of mine! She still lives around here."

"I know. I saw her recently. How did *you* get involved with Claymont?" Berry asked.

"In the 70s, most of us at Claymont had studied with J.G. Bennett, a philosopher in England. He was a physicist in the coal industry, but we had heard of him because of books he'd written on spiritual growth or lectures he'd given in the States. Actually, I hadn't read the philosophical stuff, only his autobiography. His eclecticism corresponded to my sense of there being a spiritual foundation underlying all religion. I assumed he was dead because of the dates in his book. Then a friend of mine who's a Catholic priest showed me the brochure from Bennett's school at Sherborne House."

"I'm Catholic," Berry interjected, "however, my grandfather had been invited to leave the church due to his strong opinions. Years later when I lived in New Orleans I returned to the fold—not always in tune with the orthodoxy, having more of an existential bent. Nevertheless, I'm serious about my spirituality."

I glanced again at the black-beaded rosary wound around the handle of her basket.

"So, what was Bennett's school about?" Berry asked as she fussed with her pillow, trying to find a comfortable position. "Would you put this under my neck?"

I stood up to help, but no matter where I placed the sausage-shaped cushion, she wasn't comfortable.

"Push it further down," she urged, "as far as you can." Pressing it under the upper part of her hunched back didn't look very hopeful, but that satisfied her.

When Berry was finally settled, I answered. "His school was like a co-ed monastery, though *he* never referred to it that way. I later learned that Bennett had spent time at several Benedictine monasteries. When reading about one, I discovered that the schedule and activities were similar to Sherborne's.

"It was a ten-month program," I said. "People of all ages, some older than Bennett who was seventy, came from everywhere in the world. There had been so many Americans, however, he thought we ought to try establishing a community based on the ideas he'd been teaching."

I explained to Berry that through continuous education Bennett thought humans could keep changing, developing their spirituality to become of use to the source of all creation. He said that traditional monastic life had been destructive to Western civilization by having the most spiritual of people renounce having children. I hadn't ever thought of those implications before. He suggested that Claymont also run a course like Sherborne's to prepare new community members.

"My interest in community originated when I was travelling around Europe and living with my fellow travellers. I liked the cooperative feeling and learning things from people I wouldn't have met under ordinary circumstances. Also, for years I'd thought living in a monastery was an interesting idea. Maybe because life seemed unduly complicated. It was kind of a joke, nothing I'd heard about real people doing. But remember how it was in the sixties and seventies? So many of us were excited by our new global appreciation—environmental awareness, sustainable technology, Eastern religions, the new psychotherapies."

Berry's comment was, "You're so intellectual."

"Well...maybe," I said, suddenly suspicious. Actually, I thought I was but no one else ever seemed to confirm it. Was she putting me on?

I said, "I certainly was at odds with most of my schoolmates. They didn't seem to care much about those ideas. It wasn't until I met college students a couple of years younger that I came across others who pursued the new activism. Living in the city, most of our parents were first generation Americans. I think they were baffled. They didn't know how to include us in the old ways...and they very much wanted us to fit into American society. But our interests were a little unconventional to their way of thinking. We felt our so-called 'radical' ideas were just a natural next step in our idealistic democratic education."

The Sixties

*One of the things I learned the hard way was that
it doesn't pay to get discouraged. Keeping busy and making
optimism a way of life can restore your faith in yourself.*
- ANONYMOUS

The Director of the nursing home came in, greeting Berry and her roommate and me cheerily, unloading an armful of disposable diapers into the closet. Berry, on good behavior, made pleasant small talk. "Have a nice day," she waved as the director was leaving the room. That's when Berry informed me that the woman had been checking up on us.

"We laugh too much," Berry divulged. "It's not in my treatment plan."

As usual, she had to remind me where we had left off. "You were talking about activists."

I pointed out that although all these groups had great intentions, there always seemed to be a lot of infighting and behavior contrary to the ideals we espoused. Civil rights workers vied for control of their organizations. Alternative practitioners claimed their particular therapy could cure anything. Psychotherapists encouraged patients to confront their families.

Berry and I reminisced about those gurus who were notorious for having sex with their students and bilking supporters for thousands, making them live in poverty while the teacher had everything he could possibly want. We wondered what in the world that Indian guru could do with twenty Rolls Royces. No one seemed to question the personal contradictions of leaders like him. All in all, a lot of us realized we were still lacking some important information on *how to be.*

Berry laughed. "Well, I was never involved with communities, though I heard about them, of course. I did do some civil rights work helping register voters. In Mississippi, the county we lived in was mostly black and the chancery clerk, who was the top official, was black, too. She asked me to be her deputy because she was getting so much flak—from the white community, I suppose. In our first days, we were accompanied by Dorothy Day of *Catholic Worker* fame."

"Really?" I asked, "I just recently read Day's book *Loaves and Fishes* about her work with poverty and a radical newspaper. She was a Catholic activist, sort of a self-appointed nun."

"That's her!" Berry said, "She came to stay with me while we were registering people. My dog had eaten her shoes so we had to go to town for new ones, but no one would wait on us." With a mischievous grin she added, "Our friendly attorney from Natchez had his substantial teenage son go into a store with us and loomingly suggest that the proprietor take our money."

I laughed, imagining these two women being 'protected' by a threatening teenager who towered over the store owner.

Then Berry asked me more about Bennett. I never knew what I was going to say when talking about him. It came out different every time, depending on my growing understanding and the openness of the person who asked.

"He helped me reconnect with a sense of hope. It felt as if the whole world were on the brink of a change in how us humans viewed ourselves and each other. One day Mr. Bennett talked about perceiving the same thing and how his school was a response to the time. It was confirming that someone else had the identical feeling."

"I'm not sure that I felt that," said Berry, "but I was strongly drawn to getting involved in civil rights work."

"And didn't you learn something from it? I mean, something about yourself?" But I didn't wait for an answer. "In our activist settings, we benefitted from trying to change the established order and reconcile our differences. Those efforts moved us to a new level of awareness—realizing that we ourselves created the impediments to a more peaceful existence. That was another part of what Bennett was teaching."

"I'd love to hear more about it but I'm suddenly very tired, Berry said apologetically. "It hits me like that. I need to rest now."

"I'm sorry. I hope we didn't overdo it." I *had* stayed longer than usual.

"No, please come back when you can."

I'd already begun visiting regularly by that time but I asked, "Is it okay if I come on Thursday?"

"You're so polite."

Embarrassed and amused, I giggled. "Anything you'd like me to bring?"

"Do you know what hummus is?"

That was a surprise. "Uh huh, kind of a chickpea paté."

"I love hummus. It's almost the only thing I eat any more. Usually my daughter Kathryn brings it. She's been terribly busy lately and hasn't made any. You know what the food *here* is like," Berry said, directing my attention to her tray.

I stared at the abandoned breakfast—maroon plastic dishes, white bread and instant oat meal, two cups of cold coffee (so as not to burn the patient), and scrambled eggs covered with a sharp-edged square of translucent orange cheese. A dozen packets of salt, pepper, and non-dairy coffee whitener surrounded the plate like soldiers in ambush.

Berry insisted on giving me money to buy the hummus. "Take some bills from the plastic medicine bottle in the basket. I keep them rolled up in there."

Monasteries

Those who dream by day are cognizant of many things which escape those who dream only by night.
- EDGAR ALLAN POE (1809 - 1849)

"I keep my money right here with my pills. No one would dare touch it." I didn't understand why it would be any safer there.

Couldn't they just claim they were getting her her pills? She told me to take five singles. I removed the red rubber band that was holding the tight little bundle together and fought the tightly curled bills in order to count them out.

At the grocery store they had a good brand of hummus made with olive oil, tahini, and few other ingredients. Next visit, as soon as I arrived, Berry eagerly asked about the hummus. I tried to give her the change which I had kept along with the receipt. Instead, she insisted on giving me more money so I could purchase two or three containers at a time. "That way I'll have some for the day between your visits," she explained. That's when I started keeping a running tab in my wallet—not that Berry seemed in the least concerned. I was just self-conscious about handling her money, being a new person in her life.

Berry wanted to know more about Sherborne. I told her, "I had been determined to go there, thinking it would be quiet like I imagined a monastery to be. Instead I found it very hard. I couldn't stand living day and night in the company of a hundred people. If there hadn't been so much required silence, I doubt I would have lasted more than a few weeks."

"How was it organized?"

"The whole student body was divided into three groups," I explained. "Each one alternated house duty every third day, doing all the cooking, cleaning, animal care, and maintenance. On the other days, we attended classes from early in the morning until late at night. They included a kind of sacred dance and practical work like gardening in addition to philosophy and meditative exercises. As tired as I was from our long schedule and physical activity, after everyone went to sleep I had to stay up another hour or so just to enjoy the cerebral quiet."

"Maybe that's what alcohol did for me," Berry muttered.

I didn't respond, not really sure what I thought about that. Instead I said, "Another funny thing about thinking of Sherborne as a monastery was that it turned out that the grand three-story rambling estate had actually been built around the remains of a monastery. On the first floor, there still existed a cloister and the old monastery kitchen which we still used. The stone floor had been worn smooth over the centuries and the feeling in those rooms was unique."

Berry pressed her temple with her left hand but said nothing about what appeared to be a surge of pain. Should I have asked her about it? I didn't. Surely she'd tell me if she wanted to. Then I mentioned Linda Schiller-Hanna's intuition workshop I'd gone to the year before where another image of a monastery visited me.

"Linda asked us to go to what she called the corridor of our higher self and find a door. 'Note what it looks like,' she said, 'and walk through it. Meet yourself in a past life. Ask yourself about a relevant lesson you learned in that life that you are applying in this one.'"

Berry seemed amused, smiling, no doubt, at the imaginative possibilities engendered by such an exercise.

I described to Berry what I had seen in my mind at the workshop. "The long corridor was lined with doors. Hesitantly, I walked up to a wooden one shaped like a gothic arch, carved on the surface, echoing the carved contour of the jamb. It was a form I usually think of as very grand, yet this door was small in scale, probably not even as high as a standard house door. Walking through it placed me in the cloister of a monastery. I looked around at the u-shaped building I was exiting. A covered walkway held up by columns hugged it and surrounded the courtyard on three sides. In the center, open to the sky, was a carefully tended herb garden. Approaching me was myself as a bearded monk, glowing with contentment. I understood that I was living in a protected environment. I loved prayer, feeling connected with all for whom I prayed. And the plants—each one so unique and tender. I also loved the silence of that life.

"I told me, 'You've come to your current life to bring spiritual practice into it, separate from the context of religion. You purposely chose a situation devoid of formal religion and limited family obligations so you would not be easily distracted from learning how to bring spirit into a secular life. Now it's time to take a stronger stand. Don't hang back so much. Bring that spirit to light along with others who are doing the same.' My monk-self was encouraging and enthusiastic."

Then, feeling an undisguised petulance, I added, "I told myself the experience was *just* my imagination, but what always makes me question that explanation is how true such envisionings feel. Why would that particular image come? Maybe it's true on some symbolic level. Then, I wonder, Does it matter whether it's symbolic or literal? Either way it has the same effect, doesn't it?"

Berry remained silent, allowing me to continue my monologue. "I always ask myself that. After the workshop I examined my answer more deeply. If I really believed in the literal truth of the monk experience, wouldn't knowing I lived beyond this particular lifetime give me a very different perspective?"

Maybe that was the first of many times when Berry said something like, "Oh, the pain we cause ourselves by our reluctance to believe." I don't know why I never asked her, Believe what?

Cultural Creatives

Be like Grandmother Spider
who created the world by imagining it.
- NATIVE AMERICAN WISDOM

Leaving the nursing home that day, as I walked over to the car, I jammed my cold hands into my pockets, feeling the crinkled paper money Berry had just given me. Although I'd already been visiting her for weeks, I was still questioning why. All I knew was that I'd been trying, in recent years, to be more in touch with an intuitive sense. Here was an urge with no reason and I was listening to it. With no further considering, I aimed my blue Camry toward the grocery. Two containers of hummus, coming up.

The following Thursday when I arrived, Berry was asleep. Knowing she didn't always sleep well at night, I just sat quietly and closed my eyes for awhile. It wasn't very long before she may have sensed someone's presence and opened her eyes, greeting me cheerily.

"Did you bring the hummus?" she asked and, already knowing the answer, held her hand out to receive it. However, she was unable to tear the sealed foil under the plastic lid and she handed the container back to me, watching me struggle with it. Was I going to have to go off in search of a knife? Finally successful, I rummaged around for the metal spoon she kept in her basket. It was dirty and I stood up to take it to the sink but Berry wouldn't let me wash it.

"It hardly matters in my condition, does it?" she snapped impatiently, and while I laughed nervously she added with finality, "You're kind of prissy."

A few days before, Berry had asked to see the health newsletter my husband Bruce and I had published for a couple of years. When I showed it to her I said, "This wasn't particularly his kind of subject matter, but he'd had years of editorial experience and his lack of familiarity with complementary medicine was helpful. If what I wrote wasn't clear to him, how would the readers understand it?"

The issue I chose to show her contained an article relevant to our conversation about how I'd come to study with Bennett. I said, "The newsletter's purpose was to describe the new paradigm of health care with its emphasis on mind, body, and spirit and moving energy through the person to create health. I also included the effects of environment and, especially, culture on personal well-being."

"That's a different angle." Berry said as she scooped another spoonful of hummus into her mouth.

"The article I wanted to show you," I said, "is a follow-up to the social movements of the nineteen-sixties we'd been talking about. In it I presented a synopsis of a column by P.H. Ray from *American Demographics** about the emerging culture." Berry was eating with concentration but she was listening, too.

I summarized how Ray described three world views. He called the first Traditionalism, which accounted for 29% of the American population. It's image, including small town life and strong churches, was exemplified by movies with John Wayne and Jimmy Stewart. The second view, Modernism, accounted for 47% of Americans, placing a strong value on personal success, consumerism, materialism, and technological rationality.

"That seems to cover most of American culture," Berry noted.

I agreed, nodding my head. "Now, here's something that surprised me. The third world view, Trans-modernism, was a group he referred to as the 'cultural creatives.' Preferring new experiences to new possessions, they accounted for about 24% of the population."

"That's a much bigger group than I would've thought," Berry said.

"Me, too. And he even says that they don't realize how many of them there are because they aren't given much mainstream press." I continued reading.

With attention on global issues, social conscience and activism, sacredness of nature, ecological sustainability, voluntary simplicity, self-actualization, altruism, and limited growth, the creatives took as their icon the photograph of Earth taken from outer space.

I skimmed the article, summarizing some parts and reading other sections in full. Then, concerned I might be boring her, I asked, "Should I continue?"

Berry had put aside the hummus and nodded.

Ray pointed out the irony of their not being given press since they love information, following the news and reading voraciously, although watching less TV than the other groups. Along with their general optimism was a strong orientation to holistic and alternative health practices.

Remind me to show you the *Healing Arts Directory*," I interjected. Then continuing, I read more.

What they rejected was equally interesting: hedonism, materialism, cynicism, world views based on scarcity or fear, non-ecological attitudes, and religious intolerance. Their global orientation typically included a love of foreigners and the exotic, enjoyment of gourmet and ethnic cooking, natural healthy food, and authenticity in the products they purchased.

I interrupted myself again to say, "You know, Michael Crichton spoofed this inclination in his novel, Timeline, saying that the current love of authenticity could lead to time travel being the next big entertainment industry.

After we both laughed, Berry said, out of context, "Your expository writing is so fine."

I wasn't sure how to take it. Was she teasing me? But then she encouraged me to read on.

Shortly after Ray's article, John Astin designed a survey sent to a random sample of 1,500 people on their use of alternative medicine. He wrote about the results in the Journal of the American Medical Association**. While respondents cited benefits of using alternative therapies, most curious was their agreement with a statement on the survey which was considered predictive of their use of complementary or alternative health care: I have had a transformational experience that causes me to see the world differently than before. It was found that this group was more likely to hold the values that Ray had identified as belonging to the 'cultural creatives'.

Berry said doubtfully, "Well, I'd like to think that a large segment of our culture might be feeling changed by a spiritual experience—I assume that's what they mean by transformational—but I wonder if its really true."

I didn't know either, but I was excited that Berry seemed to share my interest in the subject.

"In my life," I confessed, "it's taken a lot more than one transformational experience to see the world differently." Berry shook her head sympathetically while I explained, "I'm always struggling with doubts. I learned very young to reject spirit as something 'unreal.' The people around me dismissed any kind of spirituality with cynicism—the wittier, the better. Optimism was reserved only for the physical world—school, work, money. Without spirit, I increasingly lost interest in the physical world."

*American Demographics February 1997
**Journal of the American Medical Association May 20, 1998

Memoirs and Stories

Pronoia: The realization that life is a conspiracy
to liberate you from ignorance, flood you with love,
and give you exactly what you need, exactly when you need it.
- ROB BREZSNY

Usually I visited Berry twice during the week and once on the weekend.

"I brought three containers of hummus today," I said as I set one on the bed tray and walked around the bed to put two on the cabinet to Berry's left. "That should last you the weekend, I hope."

"Did they have garlic?" She was on a new jag.

"There was only one so I got you one roasted pepper and one basil. There weren't any plain."

Berry was already digging into the hummus while she told me some relatives visited, but she didn't say much about them. It was hard to tell whether she was happy about it or not. Indirectly expressed, the importance seemed to be about saying good-bye.

I talked about work. At FEMA I wasn't taking applications over the phone any more. Now I was working the cases—assessing what damages would be covered after inspectors had examined the property. Most everyone was disappointed with the amount of reimbursement money, but I told Berry, "If you explain how the system works, people understand that the funds available have to cover the basics of shelter for everyone with damage to their homes. All of their ruined possessions can't be replaced, although each state has specific items they will cover." After a pause I said, "It can be moving how some people are so grateful for whatever aid they receive."

A couple of times, when Berry mentioned writing memoirs, I renewed efforts to help her work the tape recorder. Eventually, we concluded it was just too awkward. "Why don't you let me take dictation?" I asked.

She dismissed my proposal saying, "I've never been able to stay focused on my thoughts when I'm dictating to another person." This was a topic we revisited several times which, finally, perhaps, because she'd gotten to know me better, Berry thought we could try.

"...but only on one condition," she added.

"What's that?" I asked warily.

"That you let me help you with your writing."

Delighted by her offer, I instantly agreed to it. I had told her I wanted to learn to write more creatively, different from the style I'd used in the newsletter.

When Berry found it easy to dictate to me she said, "It's because we think alike. Your personality doesn't divert me."

It seemed perfectly natural. When she 'wrote', I watched her as she looked up into the ether, speaking as if she were reading out of a book. She began with the thought that only "one whose eye is on the sparrow" could resolve the doubt with which she felt her memoir would be burdened.

At first break, I confessed, "I don't have a clue what that means." You could almost see her rolling up her etheric sleeves as she determined to make me more literate, explaining to me that she had been quoting the bible—that God was the one who was aware of all things, even the sparrow, and it was He who would decide the value of her writing.

Sometimes we talked about what she wrote afterwards and sometimes she prepared by telling me stories beforehand. Berry had been born in Mississippi. Her mother was an only child, the grandmother several years older than her husband. Berry described her mother as someone who took fervent control. When, as a teen, she squabbled with the young man to whom she was engaged, she quickly married a replacement. He didn't last that long either as he was young, too. Berry said, "After they had two children, he sought a more agreeable situation and wasn't seen again for some years." The babies were Berry and her younger brother Darrell.

This was going to be more fun than I had expected. I found her first forty-three word sentence utterly refreshing after two years of my newsletter's self-imposed thirteen word limit.

At first, I took my handwritten notes home, typed them into the computer, and then printed them out in 24 point type. Berry would read them when I wasn't there. Already unable to write, she would make a red mark where she planned changes. Then, when I came back, I would read the marked manuscript aloud and insert changes she dictated. She would have me read again from the beginning of the section, always remembering what we had been working on.

I resurrected my old laptop PC that was beginning to fall apart and took dictation on it using a disc. If it did fall apart, at least I'd have the material.

Many times, when I laughed at Berry's jokes, she would stop speaking and look at me with surprise. "People don't usually know when I'm being funny. It's because I'm so serpentine and you're so intelligent. You are serpentine, too," she added.

I had only a vague sense of what she might mean by 'serpentine,' uncommonly assuming it to be something good.

As Berry told it, her mother and the young husband, before he'd left her, were living on a plantation seventeen miles from her parents. While her father hunted and rode, her mother kept close company with an Afro-American 'dowager' famed as a chef of ground hog and possum cooked with wild garlic. She entertained Berry's mother with stories, intended to be made into a novel.

I didn't understand who was going to make it into a novel— Berry's mother or the dowager. Not wanting to interrupt, however, I never remembered to ask.

When Berry's mother became sick and was unable to ride her horse for two weeks, she was brought home to her parents. Berry told me, "The doctor claimed she was faking just as she had magnified her difficulties during childbirth. A second doctor confirmed the opinion."

At the time her mother's illness began, Berry was about three and Darrell a year younger. Berry later inserted a paragraph about her grandfather who gloated over his role in saving Berry's life as an infant. She had begun losing weight and would have died if he hadn't found a formula that agreed. Her grandfather experimented for weeks feeding her different foods such as lime water or gelatin. He told the story repeatedly throughout her childhood.

"It sounds like he was very devoted."

Berry snapped, "My own growing pride, however, was never diminished by *his* heroics."

Berry's unapologetic awareness of herself made me laugh. In her narrative, she described her mother's continuing weakness, weight loss, and fever. A trip to the Mayo clinic resulted in a diagnosis of chronic fatigue. She wrote that her grandfather asked what she could be tired of. Since I was pretty sure chronic fatigue hadn't become a diagnosis until my generation, I assumed she invented his comment for humorous effect.

"Grandpapa was sure my mother was going to die and despaired over God's absence, whereas Grandmama assured us that Grandpapa was just going through a normal doubting phase that God expects."

Berry always portrayed her grandfather as unsmiling and overbearing. He decided, against Berry's mother's will, to have her teeth pulled out when more logical cures didn't help her. Although this was a fairly common tactic in those times, it, nevertheless, destroyed their relationship for life.

Her grandmother, by contrast, was the family peacemaker. "Either she was oblivious or purposely hid among her literary treasures," Berry explained.

I remarked that Berry's language when she wrote was rather

different from what I was used to. "It's refreshing, and I usually understand what you're saying," I teased. She smiled.

Her ability to handle the pen was deteriorating rapidly. I kept bringing different kinds of pens hoping they'd be easier for her to hold but new problems stymied us. She could no longer get the cap off or separate one page from another. That's when she first mentioned that her agreement with the nursing home did not allow them to feed her.

After a couple of weeks of working on the memoirs, Berry wanted a break. She sharply rebuffed my prodding her to continue.

"I'm thinking," she said. "I write a lot in the middle of the night. When I have more material, I'll tell you." Then, pointing me in a new direction, she suggested, "Now would be a good time to work on one of your stories."

I was eager and had already chosen one. I told her about it that day.

"Years ago, when I was in Greece, I met an American sailor who was a twin. We were both taking a small boat that brought crew and visitors out to the *Independence*, the aircraft carrier. Do you remember it?"

Berry nodded.

"It was stationed outside of Athens in the late sixties," I continued. "A few of us American tourists met a group of sailors in a cafe. When we discovered most of us were from Chicago, they invited us to tour their ship.

"On the way out to it, there was this sailor—not part of our group—maybe returning from leave. We just happened to be sitting next to each other in the skiff. Anyway, we both had this compelling urge to connect. It was a feeling he had something special to tell me and that I'd better not miss the opportunity."

As I proceeded with the narrative, I leaned toward Berry, clenching my stomach muscles in anticipation of her reaction. By the time I finished talking, my belly ached.

Observing my intensity, Berry remarked, "I think if you write this up, you'll find your voice."

Writing Literature

We are confronted with insurmountable opportunities.
- WALT KELLY, FROM "POGO"

As soon as I entered Berry's room, I said, "I brought the story I told you about last time. It's very short, just a couple of pages."

Most of the vignettes I'd written throughout my life were about death. I was a little self-conscious about the topic but, actually, Berry was the perfect person to talk with about them. She had no resistance to the topic. Maybe she'd find my stories useful. They intimated the existence of an afterlife, though I, myself didn't quite believe in it.

I said to her, "I don't understand what's missing from them. Every now and then I take one out and polish it up, but they only seem to be getting worse."

"Let me hear this one and we'll make it into fiction."

"Fiction?" I asked.

"You know. Literature."

Before hearing it, she already knew what might be wrong.

When I finished reading the story to her, the first comment she made was, "That could be at least eight pages long."

"I can't imagine how to stretch it out like that. Where would I start?"

After a long silence, Berry simply proposed a different first line. Instantly, I countered with my own 'truer' version. Then she added several more lines, again stimulating my own rendition. I went home that day with enough inspiration to proceed working on my own. Getting more words to flow was difficult at first. I'd spent years practicing what I thought to be objective brevity. The habit left me with little beyond the bare bones and none of the detail that makes writing come alive.

Berry would have me read each revision, changing a word or sentence here and there, questioning my meaning, or showing me how to move the story along. In one version I changed the whole story to present tense, feeling proud of discovering how to make it all seem more immediate, but, then, it also created complications. There were memories of the past. I began to get confused about what needed to remain in the past tense. And there were descriptions of future events that shouldn't have come up yet. After getting myself thoroughly muddled, Berry put my feet back on the ground by suggesting I reinstate the past tense.

"We can experiment with tense later on. It's a good exercise," she said, always encouraging. I was willing to do whatever she suggested. I'd been writing for over 40 years and hadn't yet told these stories to my own satisfaction. Any change was research now.

In one of the early drafts, I described a sunny day in a cafe filled with tourists and then moved quickly into a story the sailor told me on the way out to the ship.

Berry interrupted me. "Was that really how it was?" she asked. "A perfect sunny day with no sense of foreboding?"

I told her that I didn't know if I'd call the feelings I had foreboding. I just had a lot of fear all during this trip. I'd always been afraid in Chicago, so I was even more fearful in Europe—afraid to travel alone, afraid to be in foreign countries. My fear seemed to come mostly from inside, yet Greece felt different from the rest of Europe. I couldn't understand or read the language at all. Even the head gesture for 'no' was to raise the chin. At first, it looks like a nod. They'd gesture 'no' at a kiosk and I'd stand there waiting to be given what I'd asked for and then they'd just stand there staring at me. It was unnerving—took me awhile to catch on, even after I was told. Another time we all held our hands up to mean 'wait' when we were about to move our van. Our Greek-American friend excitedly informed us during that delicate moment it was like we were swearing at them. In small towns, people seemed afraid to be seen talking to us. It was even worse on Crete. A man we were questioning about lodgings at first fidgeted nervously, then looked around warily, finally becoming tearful over his inability to get away from us without seeming rude. In addition, I'm kind of afraid of water, so going out to the ship was scary, too.

After telling Berry this, she scrutinized my face, looking up at me from the bed. After a long silence she said, "You need to include some of that information. It'll help set the mood."

At first she urged me to describe everything in more detail. Later, she had to rein me in, trying to help me experience how too much information diverted the story. It was all new and vague to me. Also, I was surprised, maybe even enthralled, by what came to mind simply by putting my attention on this long past event.

After several drafts, Berry brought up the subject of finding a title. I figured that must have meant I was getting close to finishing!

I ventured some titles: "*Death Twins. Twin Spirits. The Visit.*"

"No!" she said adamantly. "Something more to do with the actions of the story."

What? I thought. Didn't these have to do with the story?

We discussed a number of ideas—how sometimes we receive messages in mysterious ways, the nature of death, how people often don't believe their own experiences, emotional attachment, serendipity—finally resulting in the working title, *Carrier*. Although Berry had thought of it, she still expressed doubts.

But I liked it. "*Carrier* states the physical destination and also imparts the idea of messages conveyed—even if they might be of doubtful value."

After twelve drafts, Berry announced, "It's finished. At least for the moment," she said, warning me with a sidelong flash of her eyes. "Read it to me one more time."

The First Story—Carrier

In contemporary life we do whatever we can
to deny intuition of the invisible realms.
We clog up our senses with smog,
jam our minds with media overload.
We drown ourselves in alcohol or medicate ourselves
into rigidly artificial states with antidepressants.
Then we take pride in our cynicism and detachment.
Perhaps we are terrified to discover that
our "rationality" is itself a kind of faith, an artifice,
that beneath it lies the vast territory of the unknown."

- DANIEL PINCHBECK

Carrier

Sitting in a cafe in Athens, I was taking in the sunlight and watching cheery tourists milling about. Still, the atmosphere seemed tinged with danger, maybe because of what I'd heard about the dictatorship there. The others appeared to be comfortable. Steve and I were talking with a couple of younger tourists. The cafe was crowded—everyone dragging back packs. In addition to Americans, there were Brits, Aussies, and English-speaking Germans. To the Greeks, we were all hippies.

While everyone was talking casually, I began thinking how often my father warned me about the dangerous world. Newspapers and TV seemed to support his view. After all, we lived in Chicago, notorious for its violence. Riding the bus and el daily to the Art Institute in the heart of downtown where I went to college, provided plenty of training on how to watch out. Exposers. Pickpockets. Perverts. Nevertheless, Dad would read me the headlines of the latest crimes, hoping to keep me safely at home. Had I taken this trip in an attempt to work through my accumulated misgivings?

Always lurking as a more subtle sense of danger was the fact of being a first generation American Jew. All four of my grandparents had fled pogroms in the old country shortly before the first World War. My cousins and I overheard whispered stories about what occurred more recently in Germany—where Jews thought they were protected by living secular lives.

Why did I still feel anxious so many years later when, despite my distrust of people, casual travelling companions behaved like friends? Someone always showed up at just the right moment to point out the train station or invite me for a meal. These daily gifts should have inspired me to change my expectations of the world.

Interrupting my reverie, a group of American sailors burst into the cafe. I could hardly tell them apart with their uniforms and buzz cuts. They were so fresh and young looking, too. Their happiness in discovering us Americans transformed the chatter into a single conversation.

When several of us determined we were from Chicago, we began reminiscing about the lake, the loop, Frank Lloyd Wright. After living there so long with a sense of mortal danger, now I was having such warm feelings of nostalgia and even comfort in sharing these familiar memories.

Soon, we fell into talking about other aspects of being travellers in a foreign country. "I hadn't seen anything in English for so long," I confessed, "that when someone showed me an issue of *Time*, which I'd never before had an interest in, I read it from cover to cover, even the ads."

Inevitably, the talk turned to food. "Don't you love the fresh cooked vegetable dishes they serve in the tavernas?" asked one girl. The hum of agreement was cut short by a more pressing litany of what we missed. Hamburgers! Hot dogs! French fries! People called out favorites from where they were sitting. Hershey bars! Each mention was punctuated with a great "mmmm" as if it were, "Amen".

Before long, the sailors made a surprising offer. How would we like to tour their aircraft carrier, the *Independence*? Meet them tomorrow.

Maybe sensing some hesitation, they lured us with seductive promises of peanut butter! They wouldn't just feed us some. In conspiratorial tones, they revealed that they would give us jars to take away! They were laughing. They must have had their fill. We planned to meet them. After they left, I began wondering if I should have agreed to go. It would be great to see planes take off and land. Still, I worried, would we be able to get out to the ship and back safely?

At 10:00 in the morning, we showed up at the harbor where our sailor guides were waiting. The group of us—with me standing on the periphery—got ready to board a large motorized skiff. It was shaped like a rowboat but its scale made us appear to be miniature people. The sailors told us enthusiastically that the trip out to the ship would take about twenty minutes. The *Independence* couldn't come in any closer because of its enormous size. It's a floating combination skyscraper and airfield, one sailor bragged.

About twenty of us were able to fit into the bobbing skiff comfortably. Looking at my companions for signs of anxiety, I saw none. In addition to our eager hosts, other passengers appeared to be exhausted sailors probably returning from leave and their civilian relatives or friends.

We climbed aboard one by one, sitting wherever there was space. Steve squeezed in next to a pretty girl. I sat next to an unknown sailor whose name I learned was Jack. As we settled in, a mounting tension developed between him and me. It felt as if we'd been introduced by a mutual friend and then suddenly abandoned. We made tentative forays into conversation until he, like a fisherman in a trout stream, threw out an irresistible line, "I had a twin brother killed in Viet Nam...."

Why did he bring that up? I'd always been curious about twins and their connections to each other. How should I ask?

"When he died, did you have a feeling...?" My barely formed question opened floodgates. He hurriedly told me how he had been sitting quietly in the living room one evening. His folks were out late and he was enjoying reading undisturbed.

Turning to me he said, "Suddenly my twin brother George

was standing in front of me. He came out of nowhere. I bolted upright in my chair. 'How did you get home?' I asked him. 'What are you doing here?'"

"I've come to say goodbye," George told him.

Shocked, Jack said he lowered his voice and began speaking slowly. "You see, his nearness was so real. I was afraid I'd break the spell. I wanted to stretch time, make it last. We started to talk about stuff we did growing up. All along, I was sensing that we were talking around our feelings for each other. I was vaguely aware of emotions fluttering through my body like leaves in a breeze. I couldn't name them—until I knew I wanted to put my arms around him. But, before I could, he was gone."

Jack said he was left shaken, wondering what in the world had just happened. Had he fallen asleep? He was sure the experience was real but the clock showed that not even five minutes had passed.

"At first," he said, "I wandered around the house. Then it was as if I had become disembodied and watched myself checking the locks on every door and window."

Suddenly, he was very tired. Before falling asleep and barely knowing how he had gotten there, he realized he was undressed and in bed.

The next day, still dazed, Jack said he talked with his parents over breakfast. He described to them the reality of his brother's visit the night before. They let a long silence follow. His father, a military man, finally spoke and broached the idea of Jack visiting the doctor on base, just to check things out. Several times during the day, Jack overheard hushed discussions. Later, his parents let him know that an appointment had been made for him. He said that when they told him that, he felt angry and betrayed. Nevertheless, he went. The psychiatrist offered him tranquilizers—no words of wisdom, no challenge or false explanation. For days, he walked around in a fog, as if he'd been in a bad accident.

The following week, as he looked out the window at

home, a military car pulled up. Before the officers made it to the front door, he called to his mom and dad to come downstairs. Then the official government message was delivered—the time and date of George's death. It matched. They handed over a flag folded in the traditional triangular shape and a small package with a few possessions.

Later, he tried telling the story at several different times to friends.

"You must have fallen asleep and had a nightmare," or "Maybe the shock of the news ..," people said. For years, he was too pained and disappointed to ever talk about it again.

From the time I had sat down next to him, Jack said he had felt compelled to tell me this story. At the same time, I had felt an urgency to hear what he was going to say. Now, with the story divulged, the tension between us was gone. In its place was a new feeling of intimate joy. We sat with it.

Startled by a shadow, we looked up to see the looming carrier. Uh oh, we'll have to say goodbye. Grasping hands, we both seemed to have the same thought and fell into each others' arms. It was like being in Love, but not with anyone. I didn't want to let go.

Maybe I should hold on to him—ask for his address or something. We might never see each other again. But then, I yielded to the moment. It was all right. We wouldn't see each other again. We didn't need to.

-end-

For the first time, after making so many changes, Berry had allowed me to read the entire story without interruption. Lest I feel too content, however, she said, "Okay, we should let it sit awhile and look at it again in a few weeks."

I basked in the triumph of success. I'd told the story and gotten the page count all the way to six!

Alternatives

The very least you can do in your life
is to figure out what you hope for. And the most you can do
is live inside that hope. Not admire it from a distance
but live right in it, under its roof.

- BARBARA KINGSOLVER

Another day I lamented, "I don't understand why I find it so hard to make up a story. All I've been able to write are those true stories."

"Oh, it's easy," Berry declared. "Just look around you. Imagine what could be going on in any situation or say what you'd like to have happen."

"I've never done that. You make it sound so simple."

Still, I felt mystified by the process she described so casually. As I drove home, I tried to create something out of our own situation.

A woman unknown to a family visits their matriarch in a nursing home. Although she appears somewhat normal, she has a small braid of long hair at the nape of her neck while the rest of her curly hair is cut short. Is she to be trusted?

I never told Berry the idea. It seemed so lame and obvious. Also, the thought occurred that I might make Berry fearful of me. I wondered how Kathryn felt about my being there. Besides, I was still trying to rationalize my visits.

We never did get around to looking at *Carrier* again, our minds always moving forward with new material we hadn't yet shared. When I could quiet myself long enough, I realized that our reminiscing was making me feel as if I were pulling files out from some dusty cabinet, discovering what I'd saved over the years. If I were going to keep them, might there be a different way to organize them?

They weren't the old familiar collection of angers and disappointments. The newly persistent topics were mysterious events that engendered optimism, not rage. Habitually having put them on the back burner, talking with Berry brought them to the fore, along with a fleeting but increasing sense that only they, of all my experiences, were of ultimate significance, harbingers of a truth I was still striving to understand.

Yet these short-lived contemplations were repeatedly drowned out by my ongoing concern with work and personal projects I hoped would initiate the discovery of my true vocation. I was scrambling to finish the *Healing Arts Directory* for publication when I brought an old issue of it to show Berry.

"It's a local guide to alternative health care practitioners," I explained. The people in the Shenandoah Alliance for the Healing Arts thought a directory would let the community know that all these practitioners were out here and also provide some information about different therapies. I had volunteered to do it because I knew how and had already written articles that could be modified for use in it. Unfortunately, the fees for advertising barely covered the costs of printing, computer upkeep, and the time it took to do layout and distribution.

"How had the Alliance come together?" Berry asked.

"We all met through one of the events sponsored by the Healing Arts Council I've told you about. So many practitioners came to the presentation by Lewis Mehl-Madrona, a Native American M.D., that we decided to create an informal network for getting to know each other."

Then Berry said quietly, "Oh, I'm very interested in alternative medicine. I cured myself of cancer using the Max Gerson method."

"What?!"

"Do you know about the Gerson diet?" Berry asked.

"Isn't it a juice diet?"

"...fresh vegetable juices, high potassium, low-salt, and coffee enemas for de-toxification," she explained.

"I read some impressive stories but I've never met anyone who's actually used it."

"It happened just after we'd moved up here and I'd begun working in D.C. When we were still in New Orleans we thought I had pneumonia. I ran a temperature and was somewhat delirious. The doctor put me in the hospital. Kathryn was little then and, thankfully, he let her stay with me on a cot in my room. I had asked her to bring a book with her so she could read to me. Unfortunately, she chose *Mein Kampf...*"

I exploded in laughter, imagining her business-like little girl, pony tail gathered primly at the nape of her neck.

Berry shook her head. "She was a prodigy—read to me night and day, constantly asking me the meanings of the big words. My doctor had gone on vacation and his substitute actually turned his back to me and covered his ears when I tried to talk with him. I was so angry that I signed a blank check and went home."

She added, "Apparently, the combination of antibiotics and Hitler got me well enough to make the escape. But I still hadn't stopped coughing. It would often take a few minutes to get those racking coughing spells under control. When my regular doctor returned from vacation, he came to my house to tell me about the x-rays. They showed a crab-like mass in my right lung which he was sure was cancer. He wanted me to get biopsies from a specialist back in New Orleans, you know, let them interfere by cutting me open and making it worse."

I sympathized with Berry's assessment of that method of diagnosis.

Berry said she had worked for a doctors' office in D.C. where they specialized in cancer treatment. "That's what convinced me not to go that route. They'd operate or use radiation—always something invasive—and never do anything to change the person's diet, just told them to go home and eat plenty of meat and potatoes."

"How did you learn about Gerson?" I asked.

"I met a man on the train going in to D.C. who was an environmentalist. When he heard my story he suggested we go to the Library of Medicine together. We spent days looking over Dr. Gerson's lectures and articles, getting them translated into English. I did everything Gerson suggested except for one thing." She smiled mischievously.

I looked at her askance. "What was that?"

"I kept drinking. Even so, I got cured. It only took a few months," she added nonchalantly.

I was about to speak but changed my mind. Since Berry hadn't let them take tissue samples, there wasn't any proof it had been cancer. We both knew the scientific angle. Whatever it was, Berry *had* finally gotten better.

I asked her if she knew that Gerson's daughter had been running a clinic using her father's treatment techniques. Berry's face fell. "I heard that the daughter's partner had swindled her out of it." I wasn't aware of that, nor did Berry know anything more. However, she gave me an assignment, something that would occur many more times during our relationship.

"Read *Death Be Not Proud* by John Gunther. It's a small volume. He was a journalist who wrote about his spirited teenage son who was dying of brain cancer and how Gerson's diet put it into remission for awhile."

I asked, "Have you heard of the Cancer Control Society?"

Berry shook her head.

"At their annual conference, they conduct tours of clinics in Mexico—one of which uses Gerson's treatment. I thought it was his daughter Charlotte's. Also, as part of an informational package you can purchase from the Society are lists of names and phone numbers of people who have undergone therapy at those clinics. You can phone them and talk with them about their experience. It's great support for people who choose non-conventional treatment."

"You should be teaching people about these things," Berry said emphatically.

That's what I had been trying to do with the newsletter. I just needed to find the right way to do it. I wasn't a famous practitioner, nor did I have credentials that would allow me to tell people what to use for their conditions. The longer I wrote about therapies, the more convinced I became that illness comes mostly from the attitude we have about how we spend our waking hours. What people want regarding health care is to get rid of their symptoms, not an education.

Child's Eye View

One of the problems of taking things apart and seeing how they
work—supposing you're trying to find out how a cat works—
you take that cat apart to see how it works,
what you've got in your hands is a non-working cat.
The cat wasn't a sort of clunky mechanism
that was susceptible to our available tools of analysis.
- DOUGLAS ADAMS, HITCHHIKER'S GUIDE TO THE GALAXY

After we completed our first foray into my writing, Berry was ready to continue with her memoirs. The day we started on them again, after dictation, she hungrily ate the hummus I brought. She didn't usually wait that long to get at it; breakfast must have been okay. When she finally put the hummus aside, she told me what a challenge her little brother Darrell had been.

"He would never go along with my stories, always wanting to get to the facts. It annoyed and disappointed me when he did that but, no doubt, it was the beginning of his career in law. I was always proud of him when he pinned down *other people*."

"It sounds like he was so serious."

"He was, and I loved him. He begged everyone to help him learn to read and after he could, I felt like he was lost to me."

"Why?" I asked, suspecting his preference for nonfiction.

"It was the end of our communication. He chose books over me."

Berry said her mother's health continued to decline. She seemed to have no interest in anything, including their cook Charlotte's chocolate cake. She cried silently and refused to see anyone. A decision was made to send her to Colorado Springs where she might benefit from the mountain air. Berry, only seven, and apparently as precocious as her daughter Kathryn turned out, was sent along as caregiver.

She said, "One of the porters asked if I were the nurse and when I answered in the affirmative, he declared they would have to mind me, which, of course, I thought appropriate."

I found Berry's childhood confidence an entertaining contrast to my own fearfulness and the concomitant frustration it caused in the people around me.

The next time I saw her I said, "I put no stock in the *tabula rasa* theory."

"Me neither." Berry was already prying open the container of hummus. "Ah, garlic today." I enjoyed her anticipation of it.

"Who was it," I asked, "that thought babies come into the world with their minds like a blank slate, undetermined in behavior until the experiences of life make their marks? Descartes?"

Berry nodded, "A man's theory," she mumbled as she dug around clumsily for the spoon in her basket. "Just ask any mother with several children. She'll tell you how different they are."

I disentangled the spoon from the over-burdened basket and handed it to her.

"A neo-natal nurse I was talking with," I said, "noticed that when certain infants cried, it aroused extreme tenderness in her. She wanted to soothe and protect them, while another baby's crying might just irritate her. When she observed herself having these two reactions within minutes, she didn't think she could blame it only on her own mood."

Between mouthsful, Berry said, "See? Even newborns affect the adults around them differently. And when the kids are a little older they can be downright manipulative and mean. They certainly aren't always as innocent as they're made out to be."

To confirm what she was saying, I told her, "As a child, I remember working hard, practicing holding onto anger and choosing revenge, making mean-spirited decisions without understanding the consequences. Right into adulthood, unfortunately. It kept me from moving on to what might have worked better in life. Eventually, I realized I had wasted years that could have been spent more profitably contributing to my welfare." After saying that, I felt a sharp sadness and added, "I guess I needed a long lesson before realizing I could choose other possibilities."

Maybe it was our conversation about children that fueled

Berry's dictating a story about her own childish manipulation. It had occurred when she and her mother were still new to Colorado.

"I thought it would be a fine thing if there were a little girl who lived across the street who was going to give a party."

"You mean there wasn't one?"

"That's right. And I talked about the festivities to myself in a quiet tone, just dreaming up my story. Mama overheard and ordered Edna, our caregiver, and me downtown to buy me new party clothes. She instructed us not to buy pink because it didn't look good with my skin. I immediately checked it out in the mirror to confirm the error of her perception."

My laughter interrupted her. "You always laugh at my jokes," Berry told me once again, "No one else does. They usually don't even know I'm making them."

It made me feel special that I knew she was making them when others didn't. It felt a lot better than being asked what I was laughing about. That's what usually happened when I unwisely assumed people knew they were being funny.

She continued. "When we arrived back home with a fancy dress, shiny new shoes, and fresh white underclothing, Mama asked when the party was. I didn't want to put these treasures away, so I said it was that afternoon at 4:00, a time she had often proclaimed to be the perfect visiting hour.

"At the appointed time I went across the street and knocked on the door. Surely Mama and Edna were watching me. Would there be any children living there? It was a long time before the door was slowly opened and only a crack. A hunchbacked man with a huge head told me that no children lived in his house. I had to come up with a story for Mama fast."

I blurted, "Oh, my God, If I had tried something like this I would've been weeping and confessing my sins to my parents long before it had gone this far."

Berry looked proud, her eyes twinkling. "I told Mama that the dear child had been killed in an auto accident."

Again, I burst out laughing, admiring Berry's audacious efforts to control her life.

"Mama wanted to take flowers over. I terminated that possibility quickly, saying the father told me they weren't having any visitors."

I didn't notice anything in particular about Berry's use of language when she was talking to me like this. Yet her writing continued to sound unconventional. Perhaps it was her age—a different era. Or was it her being from another region of the country? It sometimes caused confusion but also added to the humor. When we finished discussing what she had dictated that day, she asked me what my childhood had been like.

"I remember mostly crying and feeling fearful—somehow managing to feel orphaned while I was living with both of my parents and a brother. I felt abandoned and desperate for support," I said. "By contrast, you were so independent."

When it was time for me to leave, Berry asked me to mail a few pages of the memoir to her brother, hoping for but not seeming to expect a response.

"He always accuses me of making things up," she said. "We seem to have totally different memories of what went on at home."

A Door Opens

Man is what he believes.
- ANTON CHEKHOV

A couple of months into my regular visits with Berry, the elements of my life felt once more like the shifting shards of glass in a kaleidoscope. FEMA had so many disasters that those of us on job-share were called back full-time and all the cubicles were noisily packed with extra phone workers placed between us. It was so loud, I couldn't hear my own voice. The normally comfortable work became exhausting. Furthermore, I had been using the time from job-share to complete the *Healing Arts Directory*. Now how was I going to finish it?

As when I'd first been introduced to Berry, I was again anxiously driving to work day after day in freezing rain on the mountain road. I said to her, "I foolishly discussed with my supervisor taking an occasional day of sick leave or accumulated annual leave. It was carefully explained to me that leave was for doctor appointments or physical illness, not for bad weather. So, if I crashed my car and was hospitalized, that would be okay. As long as the illness couldn't be called mental. No wonder everyone there is sick so much," I railed. "Being physically ill is endorsed! Meanwhile, we aren't allowed to attend to the real causes of our dis-ease."

Berry laughed as she pointed out, "Your deficiency in being able to play the game is an example of being 'serpentine'—honesty in ways that are not acceptable."

At least she understood it was honesty. I moved on to telling her about the anxious dreams I'd been having. "In one of them, I am stuffing my mouth with chocolate chips while repeating an affirmation intended to decrease my taste for sweets. Then, walking out on a road, I realize I haven't the slightest idea which way to go. I've lost all sense of direction.

"In last night's dream, my car spins out of control, sliding backwards as I round an icy curve. I tense up waiting for the impact. At the last minute, the car rights itself with no damage and no one hurt."

In no way did I connect my anxiety with what seemed to be a much-needed bit of good fortune—receiving a phone call from Tri-State After-Care, where I had applied to work the previous year. "It might be the answer to a prayer," I said. "It's in the next state but no further away than FEMA is. As a licensed social worker I'm to connect patients to services that could assist them when they've become home-bound after having been in the hospital."

After the job interview, Berry wanted a report.

"Their office was very busy," I explained, "and the interview strangely vague, not really asking much about my background nor telling me anything more about the job." Unwisely, I didn't elaborate, probably because I had already decided I wanted the job.

Hulda, the director, had a cubicle of her own while the rest of the room was filled with desks including one near Hulda for Cecilia, the office manager. The ambience didn't seem all that good, but, rather than give it any credence, I attributed the feeling to unfamiliarity.

From halfway across the room, I could hear Nicole, the current social worker who was going to provide training. Her congenial voice rose above the bustle of chatting nurses, therapists, and aides. Explaining something to a patient over the phone, she concluded brightly, "Well, that's a plan then." After hanging up, she joined us to be introduced. A tall neat woman probably in her late forties and sparkling with tasteful jewelry, she made it clear she was looking forward to her long-awaited departure.

Two days later, I was offered the half-time job for twice the pay of my work at FEMA. Thinking aloud to Berry, I said, "If I take my accumulated annual leave, I'll have just enough time to complete laying out the *Healing Arts Directory* before starting the new job." Then I added, "I actually have mixed feelings about leaving. My co-workers at FEMA have a refreshing quirkiness I haven't seen since the students at the Art Institute. I'll also miss the daily walks with my cheerful teammate, Pat, up and down the hills at break-time and eating fresh raspberries from the bushes on the sides of the road in the summer."

As a final bittersweet gesture, the team gave me a surprise going-away pot-luck luncheon.

"We're so happy you're leaving, we thought we'd celebrate," they teased. Everything seemed to be right on track.

Portents

Think 'impossible' and dreams get discarded,
projects get abandoned, and hope for wellness is torpedoed.
But let someone yell the words 'It's possible,' and resources we
hadn't been aware of come rushing in to assist us in our quest.
- GREG ANDERSON

At the same time I was preparing for my new job at Tri-State After-Care, I was still trying to figure out how to continue counseling, make use of the recent training in hypnosis, and schedule teaching some classes about alternative health care.

"I'm negotiating for office space to see clients and writing up workshop and class descriptions for teaching in continuing education programs," I told Berry. I had a vague awareness of my eyebrows wrinkling in worry, but managed, as usual, to brush the disquiet aside. "Also, the Healing Arts Council is preparing for its next event—a presentation by sister Anne, a nun/humorist. An earlier date had been canceled due to her becoming ill. Now, we've rescheduled the two-day event for the week before starting my new job."

Berry listened. Then she said thoughtfully, "You're trying to do too many things at once."

When I told her what I was supposed to be doing in my new job as social worker, she gave me one of her sidelong glances and waited for my full attention. "I've noticed that most social workers ask intrusive questions." When I didn't say anything, she went on. "They do it," she quipped, "to make the job more fun."

Over the next month I had a series of misfortunes. The week before starting the new job, a young man rear-ended my car at dusk, totalling it, though neither of us was hurt. I had just spent $1200 on mechanical repairs. All that money wasted. Now, I was going to have to use a rental car to make home visits. Hadn't I dreamt about spinning out of control?

A neighbor had witnessed the accident. "He should have been

able to stop easily," she said, "but he just kept right on going. He was looking behind him as he passed a car on its right."

The first patient at Tri-State After-Care was a middle-age man with emphysema. He smoked and really wanted to quit, hoping to remain as independent as possible. Nicole wanted me to convince him to go into a nursing home. Following our visit to him, she warned me never to consider using hypnosis in working with any of the patients. "Don't even mention the idea in the office. Cecilia will do whatever she can to discredit us."

I soon learned that most of my job was paperwork. Doing it correctly, according to Nicole, meant protecting ourselves from Cecilia. Almost all of the assistance given to patients by the social worker was in finding resources for the continuous flow of drugs the doctors prescribed. Additional paperwork was required by Medicaid and Medicare, each of which offered different related services—nursing home placement, sometimes equipment.

One ancient patient who, according to hospital criteria, had to be sent home, was still having blackouts and had no relatives or helpers to care for him. When Nicole saw the troubled expression on my face, she said to me, "Do not resist."

Two days later the patient was back in hospital, having been found unconscious by a neighbor. Meanwhile, Cecilia escalated challenging our every decision while Nicole spent increasing amounts of time planning war maneuvers against Cecilia.

My quickly sinking confidence at work contrasted peculiarly with the increased personal dignity I felt in Berry's company.
When I talked with Berry about the After-Care patients' distressing situations, she shook her head.

"Sometimes God uses terrible methods to make us realize his presence. There's really only one prayer that we ever need, 'Thy will be done.'"

Why should suffering make us aware of His presence? Shouldn't it be just the opposite?

My anxious dreams did not abate.

I am looking out a window at a small patch of sky between mountains and trees. At first, I see a dark stormy sky with the sun shining through cloud breaks. Then I see a bright white cloud lit up by sheet lightning. I point it out to my companion. We realize there's fire out there, at first far away, but quickly moving closer. There are heat waves directly outside. Suddenly, we know we will soon be engulfed by flames. I am totally panicked. There is nowhere to run and hide. It will be a fearsome death and I howl, "I don't want to die!"

I had a hard time accepting I'd have to buy a new car and not much luck finding what I wanted nearby. Thinking I'd have to go further in toward Washington, D.C., I guiltily delayed getting started the day I intended to go.

Over the phone that morning, a friend from the Healing Arts Council, reprimanded me, "Tell the universe what you need and then let go. Stop fretting!" Just after a calming meditation and putting my coat on, the phone rang. It was one of the local car salesmen I'd talked with the previous week.

"A trade-in just showed up," he said. "It's exactly what you're looking for and the price is lower than what you'd expected to pay. The owner is an old customer of ours. We have the full repair history. He kept it spotless. We're still going to detail it but I want you to see it beforehand."

The '93 Toyota was a golden beige color I'd recently been admiring. I drove it to Berryville where Ray, a local mechanic, looked it over and test drove it. He proclaimed it to be a great deal and when I tried to pay him, he wouldn't accept any money.

Grace

There is no remedy for love but to love more.
- HENRY DAVID THOREAU

With one problem solved, another quickly took its place. Gracie, my beautiful gray and champagne tortoise shell cat, had begun sleeping a lot more than usual and I was able to feel a lump at the top of her right front leg. She had already been limping for two years. Neither I nor the local vets ever found any reason for it, though we carefully examined all her joints and toes. For two years the homeopathic vet prescribed according to her symptoms. The limp had never gotten better or worse, although the remedy seemed to help her mood and energy level.

Now, with the appearance of the lump, the local vet diagnosed it as a fibroid sarcoma tumor. "Sometimes we can extend the life of the cat or dog for a little while,' he said, "by amputating, but the long threads of this kind of tumor always allow it to grow back. In Gracie's case the tumor is too high for amputation anyway. I'm sorry to tell you this. The animal usually doesn't live more than a couple of months after diagnosis."

I'd probably been given two years of Gracie's presence while homeopathy had slowed the tumor's development.

A few months earlier, over the phone, I asked my friend Eka, who had been studying animal communication, if she would talk with my cats, Buster and Gracie. She had never met them and I had never told her anything about them.

According to her, Buster asserted, "While it's nice that BJ tries to be fair with us, sometimes she is a little too fair and probably doesn't realize how special I am."

When I wondered if she would ask Gracie about her limp, Eka explained after a long silence, "She's balking, She doesn't want to talk about it." I took it as forewarning.

Now, Gracie was clearly going downhill. Thinking she might not have much time left after the vet's pronouncement, I phoned Eka, again, "Can you tell me anything more about Gracie?"

"She seems very far away. It's difficult to tune in. Give me a minute," and we sat in silence awhile. When Eka spoke, she said, "Gracie isn't unhappy. She thanks you for what you've done for her, for loving her."

I blinked back sudden tears. I wanted to believe Gracie felt that way. I held her in my lap after the phone call, looking into her beautiful green eyes. I'd had never been able to capture them in a photograph. Perhaps it was because of her having been feral that she always blinked at the click of the camera.

"I love you," I told her. "You've been such a good companion. I'm going to miss you. Can I hold you when you're ready to go?"

The next morning as I was preparing for work, Gracie was restless. When I was done in the bathroom, she had just arrived. Then, as I was leaving the kitchen, Gracie had just shown up. Finally, I realized that she had been trying to follow me. I carried her to the rug near the cat door where the cats often rested, looking out at the world through the clear plastic flap.

"I love you," I told her. "Would you nap here while I'm at work?" Then I hugged her, kissed the top of her head, and hastily left.

I took a long lunch so I could go home to check on her. She wasn't on the rug. I ran to the bedroom where she often napped. Apparently, she had tried to jump up on the bed and died in the effort. I found her twisted on the floor.

Why hadn't I just put her on my lap before I went to work? She had been following me. Had she been intending to die in my arms as I had requested? Instead, I was totally preoccupied with getting to that ill-suited job. When I touched her body, she was stone cold.

Meanwhile, at work, Nicole, who, in the beginning, had been friendly enough, had begun pulling back, her silent responses to my overtures unsettling. Trying to appear less threatening, I told her more of my private thoughts.

I said to Berry, "I can't stop myself even now when the feeling of danger has become ominous."

She said sympathetically, "Oh, I've done that, too."

Each work day brought another small incident—a nurse annoyed when I couldn't meet her schedule, Nicole impatient with my not having memorized the differences between Medicaid and Medicare, disapproval of my trying to help our client stay out of a nursing home. One day Cecilia became very upset toward Nicole and me when we discovered a patient's family had spent money for personal use after it had been earmarked for nursing home costs. Their misdeed had occurred over a year before I started working there but that didn't matter.

Only my visits with Berry provided a soothing balm during this period of growing tension. Two days after Gracie died, I told Berry about a vision I'd had. "I awakened in the middle of the night. Gracie was on our bed, crouching in what Bruce and I call her bun-rabbit pose. So comforted by her presence, I atypically fell back to sleep immediately."

Setting Sights

The best way to predict the future is to invent it.
- ALAN KAY

Berry's love of language and my sensitivity to feeling led us into rambling conversations about the subtle meanings of words, each discussion like a gourmet meal.

"Isn't 'dowager' grand?" Berry asked. "So much better than 'old lady.' And, if applied to hired help, so much the finer for its intimated descriptive value and humor."

Berry often accused me of having an extraordinary vocabulary and would be haughtily gleeful whenever she found a word I didn't know. I didn't think I knew that many words.

"It's my para-medical vocabulary that deceives you," I explained.

She gave me another assignment. "Look up 'amanuensis'. You'll have to figure out the spelling, too."

I didn't remember ever hearing the word and had to create several spelling variations before coming up with A M A at the beginning. *Amanuensis—a person employed to write what another dictates.* Berry was making sure I got good use out of my new *Webster's Encyclopedic Unabridged Dictionary.*

Berry and I discussed another story she was going to add to her memoirs. It was from that same early foray in Colorado. She wanted to join the Girl Scouts and her mother found a troop led by a Mrs. Hahn from New England. Berry described the uniform in detail, including a large hat, reminding me of the charming 'uniforms through the years' I remembered seeing in the Girl Scout Handbook when I was a child.

"The landlady's son took me to the street car and told me where I was to get off," Berry said. "The girls, all in those grayish-green uniforms, met in a pleasant school with big windows. As soon as we were assembled, Mrs. Hahn gave each of us a leaf which we were supposed to draw on the blackboard. She asked me where I had lived before Colorado and what school I was attending. I knew we were supposed to be in school, not taking care of our mother, so I told her I was not attending school because I wrote for *The New Yorker.*"

"What!" I exclaimed, laughing.

"Well, my grandmother had been sending this new magazine to Mama and I'd been hearing good things about it from her. And to my way of thinking, how would Miss Hahn find out about something that was going on in New York?

"The scout leader showed up at our home and earnestly explained to my mother that I would not be allowed back until I knew what was true and what was false. My mother cordially thanked her and, after she left, told me that I should distinguish between what was true now and what might become true later."

I loved that. Either her mother was very wise or Berry saw the opportunity for a great line. All I asked though, was, "Did you ever go back?"

"Oh, no. Although my mother said I could wear the uniform around the house." Then Berry sighed. "I'm done for today."

Her usual time limit was about an hour. Over the long run, it was easy to see that her strength was waning but whenever I asked if we were working too hard, she insisted she was having fun.

"I never expected to have the opportunity to do this," she told me.

We joked about things we thought we probably would have fought over if we'd been together in her healthier days. The week before, Berry had swallowed a sip of Listerine because it was too much trouble to find a place to spit it. I had reprimanded her and she refused to let me forget this 'squeamishness.'

I said, "If you'd known me years ago, you would have thought me straight and not so serpentine, as you describe me now."

"Isn't it nice we get to bypass all that?" she asked. "Now, I can just enjoy your strong intellect and admire your knowledge of alternative medicine."

Still unsure whether Berry was teasing me, I searched for irony in her intelligent eyes, and, not finding any, decided to accept the comment at face value.

When I had gathered my belongings that day, she said, "I have a poem for you to look up when you go to the library." She hadn't forgotten her intention to make me more literate.

"It's an exquisite piece of English poetry, Francis Thompson's *The Hound of Heaven*. Do you think the library in town will have his work?"

Aside from a collection of books about the Civil War, the little private library carried mostly best selling novels and romance. I wasn't familiar with Thompson.

I said, "All I know is that I've become resigned to not trying to do research there. When I need something specific I go to a public library." Then, I added hopefully, "But, maybe it'll be in a collected work."

When I stood to leave, Berry stopped me. "You must be out of money by now. Take some more to buy hummus."

"Let's see," I said, opening my wallet to pull out the yellow post-it note with minuscule numbers written in a column. "We still have a little over two dollars."

"How do you do that—make the money last so long? Are you buying the hummus yourself? I don't want you to pay for it."

"I'm not." Berry gave me a challenging look. "Really. I have some coupons. That stretches it a bit. I'm not paying for it myself," I repeated.

"Well, one container costs more than what you have left so take some money," Berry insisted, awkwardly groping for the pill bottle that held her cash and handing it to me.

She could hardly even hold the bottle now, I noted as I snapped off the cap and unrolled the bills. Hmmm, Kathryn must be replenishing it.

"Take a ten. I don't think there's anything bigger, it's mostly singles."

I took the ten and wrote it down on my note, adding it to the total. It always felt awkward to be handling Berry's money. No one questioned me, but the situation at work was making me feel even more apprehensive than usual.

Reading

Men occasionally stumble over the truth, but most of them pick themselves up and hurry off as if nothing ever happened.
- WINSTON CHURCHILL

My husband Bruce and I had spent the morning reading the Sunday paper and leisurely strolling through the farmers' market in Shepherdstown. We enjoyed our summer ritual of greeting friends and taking in the beauty of brightly colored vegetables and flowers while doing our weekly shopping for groceries. It was already lunchtime when I arrived at the nursing home. Kathryn was there, strands of her light brown hair having come loose from the bun at the back of her head. Their movement added to the appearance she often had of rushing. She had brought Berry some hot homemade soup that smelled delicious, insisting I have some, too.

Queasy about using nursing home utensils, I was glad Kathryn had found a fresh plastic cup and spoon. The soup was excellent. If she had always cooked like this, Berry must be feeling pretty deprived since coming here. But she never said so. The three of us talked about English humor, the movie *The Wrong Box*, and Kathryn's work schedule. I excused myself as soon as I politely could, not wanting to horn in on the limited amount of time they had to be together.

During our next visit, when I told Berry I had never read as a child, she was surprised.

"I'd have thought you'd have loved reading. It would have fed your intell..."

I interrupted before she completed the sentence, "Words were so gray. I'd skip them, moving from picture to picture. Images seemed to be the only color around. Maybe I learned to take solace in things like my mother did. I loved containers, miniatures, rocks, stamps, trading cards, plants, sea shells, and shiny exotic National Geographic magazine pictures."

"You should try writing about your mother," Berry suggested abruptly.

"Whoa! That would be a story for which I have no vignette to start me off. My laundry list of complaints and self-pity wouldn't be very good reading. I'll have to think about it."

Berry smiled, satisfied her suggestion would probably be carried out.

Mom and I never had any conversations. She never played with us when we were little. What would I say about her? I always seemed to be at such odds with everything, starting with my parents. Then I dropped that line of thought, and another one replaced it instantly.

"In kindergarten, our teacher held up a card that had a circle divided into three colors, red, yellow, and blue. Each segment had the name of the color printed over it. The teacher would point to a color and ask us, 'What color is this?'"

"'How stupid!' I thought. 'All we have to do is read the name of the color.'"

"See?" said Berry. "I told you you've got a strong intellect."

"I had no idea reading those words might be unusual. You know, I never actually read through a book on my own until I was sixteen when, for some unknown reason, I was inspired to wade through *Pilgrim's Progress*, of all things." Berry chuckled. "Actually, there was another book..." I closed my eyes, watching its image slowly appear. First I had to tell her about the teacher. Mrs. Koelling taught first grade. She was as glamorous as a movie star—tall with sleek blond hair down to her shoulders and bright red lips. She was always happy to see us, her rambunctious class. We were learning how to read. One day, she put such a long word on the black board that we were stunned into silence. Nobody knew what it was.

"Try to read part of the word," she urged. "Can anyone see a smaller word in the big one?" Someone quickly said, able. Almost at the same time another yelled out, table. That was at the end. Then, a boy shouted, fort which was in the middle, and another said, comfort.

"Can you put the words together?" my teacher asked. Lots of voices were trying to say it, not all at the same time. Comfort table. Comfort table. Finally, someone figured it out. Comfortable! Mrs. Koelling was so pleased and we were having fun. She explained the idea of being able to have comfort, making the big word seem like magic to me.

At the end of a day once, Mrs. Koelling passed out a sheet of paper with printing and pictures on both sides, all going in different directions. The pictures were simple line drawings like from a coloring book. She showed us how to fold the paper in half and then fold it in half again. She pointed out where to cut on some dotted lines. It turned into a book with eight pages! We colored the pictures. The story was about a big black umbrella. It was so big that five children could fit under it. I was so excited about making a book and being able to read it that as soon as I arrived home, I searched for my mother to show her. She was reading the newspaper in her usual place at the dining room table. I ran to her and held the little book up, then proudly read it from beginning to end.

"I read a whole book!" I said, waiting for her to reply.

"So what?" she answered laconically, and turned back to her paper.

Fear of Death

I said to Life, I would hear Death speak.
And Life raised her voice a little higher and said,
You hear him now.
- KAHLIL GIBRAN

One Tuesday, after embarking on a new container of hummus, Berry said, "Officially I'm allowed my sherry only in the evening, but the pain is getting worse. Would you pour me just half a cup?" she asked, pointing to the plastic water cups on the sink.

I paused to think about giving her the sherry, finally saying weakly, "But you're not supposed to have it."

"Oh, is this like my swallowing the mouthwash?" she snapped. "You fussing over the rules of my superb medical treatment? Take a look at me. Are we talking about preserving my good health?"

She had a point there. Then I caught a thought I almost didn't notice. Maybe you never would have gotten into this condition if you hadn't drunk so much in the first place! Oh, how could I be so judgmental? I was just upset with her for posing a new dilemma. How much longer was she going to live, anyway? I went to the cupboard.

After her sip, she was ready for work. "What's your next story?" She knew I had already chosen one.

"It's also about a death—my boyfriend Joe's mother. It happened several years before I travelled, when we were still in college. Joe, his brother, his father, and I were there. We never talked about it afterward. We all reacted but I have no idea what they perceived. I don't know if they had the same experience."

"Probably not."

I didn't want Berry to be right. If we'd all had the same experience, it would have seemed like proof that it really happened. I started to tell the story. "It must have been about five years before the trip to Europe—probably the first time I seriously questioned whether death was the annihilation us sophisticated people claimed it to be."

Berry said, "You know, none of us would fear death if we believed in Spirit."

When she said that, a different image popped into my mind.

"Can I tell you another story? I haven't thought about this for some time."

Berry nodded, always curious to hear a fresh tale.

I told her this had happened about five years after I'd gone to Europe. I was visiting Wright, my boyfriend, and his family in a rural area outside of Toronto. I admired him for the unique things he liked to do, though they weren't anything I would have done— like camping in Canada during the winter or skydiving. He never urged me to, either, and I liked that. We seemed to enjoy our differences. One of the first days I was there, we spent the morning sightseeing, followed by lunch and music at a Jamaican restaurant. Toronto felt familiar, reminding me of Chicago with its many ethnic neighborhoods.

"On the way home, Wright said we'd be passing the airfield

where he skydived. 'My group is out there today. Would you mind if I jumped a few times? You'd be able to see what we do and you could go up in the plane with us if you want.'

"I didn't mind stopping there. I thought it would be fun to see. We pulled into a parking lot at the edge of an endless mowed meadow. Wright introduced me to his buddies and the teacher. It was a lovely day so I just wandered among the groups of skydivers listening to their conversations. Three or four people at a time went up with the instructor whom I scrutinized before each take-off, concluding he was overly casual. I have no idea why I made that judgment. He had to turn the propeller to start the engine. It struck me as primitive and I was glad I didn't feel conflicted about choosing not to go up. Often, I badger myself to do things I really don't want to, just because others seem to think they are a treat.

"Ellie, one of the jumpers, attracted my attention. It was as if she had static all around her—silver specs I saw in my mind's eye. And she was restless. I kept thinking I should talk with her but in my shyness I hung back. Several times, just as I was about to work up to a chat, she would hop onto the plane again for the next jump. Although she was all prepared, wearing her parachute, she returned with the plane each time, not having jumped. After the third time, I asked Wright about her.

"'She's an experienced jumper,' he said, puzzled, 'but today something is bothering her and she keeps changing her mind.'

"After two jumps, Wright called it a day and we went home while the other divers stayed on. Shelling peas, dinner with his family, TV, a lot of talk and laughter with his three loud sisters, we finally went to sleep.

"The next morning in the early mist, strangely silent of bird chatter, Wright and I walked down the long farm driveway to retrieve the morning paper. When he unfolded it, we stared at the headline. 'Plane Crash Kills Three!' It was Wright's teacher and two of his students! The engine had died and they were too low to jump. Ellie was on board.

"I couldn't stop thinking about it. She must have been sensing her death. Figuring it most likely to come from a bad jump, she hadn't been able to get herself to jump. But she kept going up, maybe trying to get past the feelings, perhaps calling it her imagination. Could I have stopped her from going? If we had talked, would she have told me, a stranger, that she was unusually nervous? Would I have suggested she go home and come back another day? Should I have?"

"Psychic," Berry said.

"I picked up on something, but I didn't know what it meant. I think this kind of thing happens a lot, but we're taught not to pay attention."

Berry said, "Maybe like all the other skills in life, you have to notice the details, then experiment and practice. How many times do we fall learning how to walk? But it's another question whether we can actually change someone else's destiny, isn't it?"

We shared another of those long silences. Then, returning to the story I'd brought, Berry pointed to it in my lap, "Read it to me."

In three pages I had described Joe's mom dying of ovarian cancer and how a mysterious event occurred the day of her funeral.

"It's an important story," Berry said pensively. "This one, too, could be at least eight pages. It happens in such a rush. I want to have a sense of it taking place in real time. As short as it is, I wonder if some of the details even relate to the point of the story. Sometimes your articulate writing keeps us at a distance. What do Joe and his mom look like? Feel like? Show me their qualities through your experience."

At the next visit, I read to Berry a description I had just written about Joe and me walking in the park. Joe kept hiding and jumping out at me playfully from behind newly planted trees that were a lot smaller than he was. I felt warmed thinking back on his humor and sweetness.

"I don't like it at all," Berry said. "It's silly. It doesn't have anything to do with the story you're telling."

She was right, yet I couldn't imagine how to show Joe's tenderness. But that made me ask myself what Berry said I needed to think about—was it relevant to the tale?

Several months had passed since I began visiting when Berry said to me, "I can feel myself getting weaker. My short term memory is worse also."

I had noticed it, too. "But your thinking is still strong," I said.

"I just hope I won't get senile before we get a story published." I was touched by the plural pronoun. She encouraged me to consider sending "Carrier" to some magazines—maybe *Fate*.

Meanwhile, my nightmares continued, more often waking me several times a night. Just a week short of completing the three month probation at the new job, I dreamed I witnessed a woman being attacked, knocked out, undressed, and then debated about by a calculating heartless woman, as if her prey were a piece of trash. I gave the attacker orders in an attempt to restore the victim's well-being and dignity.

I guess I had really been keeping a lid on my uneasiness about work but the situation soon became too conspicuous to ignore.

What Was I Thinking?

For one human being to love another:
that is perhaps the most difficult of our tasks;
the ultimate, the last test and proof,
the work for which all other work is but preparation.
- Rainer Maria Rilke

At work, I wrote up patient evaluations in pencil, fearful of inking them in before talking about them with Nicole. My response to her perfectionism was to become even more cautious than I usually was. When a new client had been almost impossible to interview

79

because of his deafness, I talked with a couple of professionals at other agencies, trying to find out where to get him a hearing aid. I knew the notes I made did not belong on the evaluation, but on a separate social work sheet. Before having a chance to meet with Nicole in two days, Cecilia phoned me on my day off.

"You have to turn in your new client's papers. Today's the last day of the month."

With reluctance, I went to the office and turned them in. The following morning, I showed Nicole the case, explaining why I needed to re-write it.

"Oh, it can't be rewritten once it's turned in," she informed me, "but we can add footnotes to explain the extraneous information."

On the next work day, a different patient's evaluation had been returned to me with a note from Cecilia telling me to fill in a section on the form we had never filled in before. I asked Huldah, the director, about this new requirement.

Instead of answering my question, she said, hesitantly, "I've heard comments that you aren't doing very well." Thinking she was about to offer some advice, I asked what the problem was.

"I couldn't say. I don't know the details." Then, a long silence.

"Well, how am I supposed to correct it if you don't tell me what it is?"

"I don't know." Another long silence.

"Well, whoever said I wasn't doing something well—would *they* tell me what I need to do?"

Huldah looked away. "Maybe this job just isn't a good personality fit. I thought it would be better for you to know this before your probation time is up."

What was she saying? When Huldah confirmed what I finally figured out was bad news, I began to cry. It seemed rather unfair. Huldah began crying, too, wringing her hands. Then she added, "I find these talks so hard."

Hard for whom? I thought, especially when I had to guess what she was saying. How ironic that what I naturally did in my real life—give referrals for health care support—was the description of this job. I felt crushed by being of so little value there. But the day wasn't over yet.

Nicole and I had an evaluation to do up on the Blue Ridge. She phoned the office instead of coming in. "Meet me at Mrs. Kopel's," she said. A shiver went up my neck.

During the interview with our cheery patient, Nicole refused to look me in the eye and met my lighthearted humor with an icy stare. What was up? As we were leaving, she said, "We need to talk. Let's meet at the parking area down the road."

It was an unpaved car park, giving drivers a place to turn around on the steep mountain. Inviting me to sit on a log next to her, she said, "I'm sorry but I have no confidence in you. I cannot back you up. In this position you are expected to be a leader and it's clear you can't be one." Then, after a short pause, she added, "You intentionally put irrelevant information in your report, trying to distract the managers from what you were supposed to be writing up regarding his hospital-related needs."

My mouth dropped open. I reminded her that it was I who had brought the imperfect write-up to her, not the other way around.

I thought back to the day Nicole asked with an edge to her voice why I couldn't remember the details about all the procedures, always having to refer to my notes. I told her how hard it had been for me in school, even as a child, to memorize, how I had cheated on tests... "Oh, you did?" Nicole interrupted, sounding like a slammed door.

"Yes" was all I had said, thinking if I was to know five crops grown in Kansas, I would list the first letter of each crop in alphabetical order or make up a memorable word and write it on my palm. In art school, I knew I wouldn't have to deal with memorizing so much. It wasn't until I was 37 that I decided to chance going for a social work degree and face the memorizing ordeal again. I *had* cheated in the past. Did it matter I hadn't for my social work license? But, it was clear I had already lost Nicole, who wasn't going to sympathetically request details. Why had I ever said anything anyway? Sabotaging myself?

Nicole wasn't done. "You also did not have an answer for a

nurse on something that you should already have known how to do." Again, I asked what it had been. She couldn't tell me, instead, grumbling, "That's the least of your troubles." She seemed to be warming up to her hostility now. "You had better hand in your resignation *to me* and then I won't say anything to anyone. If you don't, you'll have to suffer the consequences. I'll tell Huldah about your incompetence. Knowing what a gossip she is, it'll soon be spread all over the district."

Disgusted by her intent to coerce me, I snapped, "Oh, please!" then stood up and marched off to my car.

"You have until Monday to make your decision!" Nicole shouted at my back.

Amazed that she was so flagrant with her intimidation, I drove straight home to mull over what had happened. Nicole obviously didn't know Huldah had already let me go. I had no legal recourse. Before probation is over, an employer doesn't have to show any reason for letting the employee go. For the record, I may as well resign, but I wouldn't hand it in to Nicole.

On Monday, as I was preparing the letter, Nicole, still unaware of what had transpired, phoned me at home, ordering me to come into the office at 1:00 p.m.

"You will turn in your resignation *in my presence.*"

That was the last straw. I hung up on her and went directly to Huldah's office. We agreed I would resign immediately. No use torturing myself by working there another two weeks. Wasn't it ironic that instead of social work, all I had been doing was procuring drugs for people?

Protection

My soul is a Mosque for Muslims,
a Temple for Hindus,
a Shrine for Buddhists,
an Altar for Zoroastrians,
a Church for Christians,
a Synagogue for Jews,
and a Pasture for gazelles.

- IBN ARABI

I pondered what had been happening, starting at over a year ago being offered a perfect job by an old employer begging me to help him. That hadn't worked out well and luckily the job at FEMA opened up. Then, once again, I'd been offered a position that sounded perfect. It got me to leave FEMA, giving me a chance to work in my own field part-time at a salary that covered the bills. What was this with my chronic defenselessness, going all the way back to childhood?

Seeking consolation, I sat down on my bed intending to meditate. My thoughts drifted. Maybe as much as a year before, an image of a certain kind of antelope had suddenly come to mind and I imagined we had run across the grasslands together, then I seemed to become her. I understood that my fear had, at times, kept me alive. Fast and beautiful, delicate and sensitive, I was able to run anywhere, but chose to stick around living the life I thought I was supposed to.

At that time I tried to remember what the animal was called. An ibex? But when I looked it up, it turned out to be a mountain goat with similarly curved horns, not the beautiful antelope I'd seen. In the middle of the night, the antelope's correct name popped into my head, waking me up. Oryx! It had been ages since this beautiful creature had appeared in my thoughts.

Now, she was back. This time the image simply appeared.

She is just standing there looking at me. So majestic—her sleek

black, gray, and white colors as elegant and deep as a Rothko paint-
ing. She escorts me to myself as an infant. I am supposed to see
something. Then I notice a baby oryx lying on the ground before
her, fawnlike, all folded up, alert, waiting to be taken care of.

Where's Mama? it seemed to be asking.

The adult oryx begins nudging the baby to stand up. It's weak,
hungry. The adult feeds her, then gently prods her into the safety
of the herd. She wants me to see the baby getting stronger, how it
grows up, becomes part of the herd. I watch the scene dubiously.

Even if this baby were not your own, this is what you must do
for her—nurture her, the oryx says. You cannot undo what she suf-
fered but you can take her with you, care for her, give her what she
needs now and bring her into a favorable environment. You can-
not run like an antelope without taking care of that baby.

Then, as me, in my mind, I enter a pleasantly daylit room with
warm light colors and comfortable couches. I am cuddling an
infant me and playing with her. When the infant me reaches out
and grasps my finger, I experience a split second of raging mater-
nal instinct, my heart enveloping this delicate baby.

After The Fall

As spiritual beings living a human existence, we are ultimately
defined by our choices and our lives provide us with certain
opportunities to redefine and even reinvent ourselves
by looking beyond the fear and pain of a particular moment
to the possibilities of transformation and transcendence.
- STEPHEN SIMON

I phoned Linda, the woman whose workshop I had attended the
year before where we visualized the corridor of doors I had told

Berry about. Sadly I described how I had lost my job.

"You need to reframe that," she said in a serious tone of voice. Then, after a long pause, she said brightly, as if surprised by a discovery, "You've just graduated!" I laughed at how different her words felt inside my chest.

Linda added, "There's something I read recently that fits this situation...what was it?...oh, yes, now I remember, 'When you fail at something, it's because you were aiming too low!'"

Yes! Why was I working in a conventional medical setting when I did not believe it to be a place of healing? I wanted to work in a situation where there's recognition that spirit and emotion are intricately woven into our state of health. Drugs that force the body to function differently aren't treating the cause of illness. In addition, look what has happened in our culture from embracing drugs for every discomfort in life. Linda encouraged me to make a self-hypnosis tape for rebuilding confidence.

"After using it for a month-and-a-half, it should be well-imbedded," she said.

I asked her if she had any thoughts on why I had been offered jobs like After-Care, only to have it fall apart. And why do I move from project to project only to have the energy suddenly disappear?

She said, "Sometimes our helpers are checking to see if we're willing to follow the inclinations they send us. Something better is coming," she said with certainty.

I could almost believe her. But hadn't this been happening all my life? Would I ever find work I was suited to?

Berry listened to my most recent goings-on, shaking her head. Although sympathetic, she repeated what was becoming a mantra, "You should put all your attention on writing. You're trying to do too many things at once."

I had just been reading *Daughter of Fortune* by Isabel Allende, envying the idea of the main character, Eliza, who, while disguised as a male, was earning money as a scribe for gold miners. It sounded so appealing, reading and writing letters for people. I hadn't mentioned the book to Berry.

The next day when I went to visit her, she excitedly told me she had an idea for my making money.

"You should let the nursing home know that you could write for people, as you've been doing for me, taking down memoirs for their families. You could also make phone calls and write letters for them. And," she added happily, "you'd be providing such a service!"

Had Berry been reading my mind? We spent the rest of the visit designing a business card.

So excited about it, Berry, from her inert position, pursued several staff members and the Director during the week. She reported back to me, a cloud casting its shadow over her, "It's apparent the nursing home wouldn't necessarily like having someone write down what people might have to say."

Not two weeks had passed when I was offered a temporary two-day-a-week job at a library not too far away. I'd bumped into Colette, a neighbor who was working there. She had just been asked to help baby-sit her granddaughter. "My daughter needs help temporarily while she finishes taking a class."

"If you could alternate with me," she said. "that would give me the days to assist her."

I liked library work and having a whole hour for lunch allowed me to chew my food, meditate for a few minutes, and travel at a reasonable pace back to work.

When Berry's daughter Kathryn was to drive to New Orleans to visit her father for a week, she asked if I would visit her mother daily. I was surprised to hear Berry worry over Kathryn's journey. Berry, who usually sounded indifferent to the difficulties of life, even looked smaller and more frail when she talked about the impending trip.

It was then that she brought up the issue of my hair style, short except for a three-inch braid at the nape of the neck. Berry boasted she'd finally found the right word to describe it—sinister! "It's too strange for around here. Why wear it that way, anyhow?"

I don't think she would have believed me if I'd told her that a number of men and women at FEMA were wearing their hair that way. It had struck me as being strangely exotic. Why *were* we wearing our hair that way?

I laughed in response to Berry's question, thinking back to my lame attempt at a fiction story line that I'd never told Berry—about a family matriarch's unknown visitor. Now I understood it was Berry who was uncertain of me—not Kathryn. During those early visits, I'd kept seeing myself as if from someone else's eyes—someone wary. Whatever misgivings Berry might have had, she'd quickly put them aside, now referring to herself as my substitute mother, an honor I didn't take lightly.

As I worked on the story of Joe's mom, we continued with Berry's memoirs. I often wished we could use bigger blocks of time and work faster but Berry's energy determined the pace.

She made me laugh with yet another portrait of herself as a little girl. There was something alike about us but I rarely would have committed my feelings to action as Berry did. It made her so much more interesting, I thought. In this story, her father who had been gone for so long suddenly joined his wife and children in Colorado.

"He was a car salesman," she said, "about to take a female customer for a ride up the mountain road. She had a daughter my age and so I was recruited to keep little Carolyn company. I found her to be pretty, yet in possession of a poor attitude. She was not friendly and my growing fears as we swayed only feet from the rocky gorge made me resent her disregard. I concluded she must die."

My laughter, once again, interrupted Berry's story. "What did you have in mind?" I asked.

"A car crash would kill me, too, so I came up with an alternative. I'd been hearing about the death-dealing capabilities of microbes and thus pretended to lick the sole of my shoe. After illuminating for her the dangers, I dared her to do the same. She was up to the challenge and followed through with such enthusiasm that I was sure she would perish.

"Not many days later, a friend of our family fulfilled my request to be driven to Carolyn's. Her mother met us at the door and I respectfully inquired about her daughter, anticipating diabolic results. When the mother called Carolyn, I was horrified to see her bounce into the room glowing with good health."

The Second Story—Joe's Mom

The opposite of a correct statement is a false statement.
But the opposite of a profound truth
may well be another profound truth.
- NIELS BOHR

"How will I ever know when I'm finished?" I asked Berry as I brought what I hoped would be the last revision of the story about Joe's mom. "It seems like I can always change a word, improve a sentence, move a paragraph."

"Well...actually you never are. It's the fate of a writer—you just have to declare it done sometime. If you have a deadline, so much the better. And if it's published and you have something new to work on, that'll at least keep you from tinkering with it anymore. I'm the same way. Sometimes I'll make big changes, too, and then change it all back to the way it was before."

I had tried *Joe's Mom* in present tense, and although Berry wasn't enthusiastic about it, she coached me through the complications. We ended up telling something more about me than I'd intended—revealing the baffling incongruity between my lamented feeling of alienation and my seeming need to distance myself from people. I almost always made the changes Berry suggested, just to try them out. My strong opinions emerged over the truth of the actions, not the structure of the writing. I don't remember most of her suggestions. When they suited me, I no longer recognized what had come from her, but occasionally her use of a word or composition of a sentence would grate, never sounding natural no matter how often I read it. I just couldn't own it—like the way we said, "A small lawn in front and a larger one in back are bordered with colorful flowers that must be zinnias." It's the "must be". She was adamant about using it. I've still not gotten used to it although now I enjoy it's oddity as a reminder of Berry.

We'd gone over it a dozen times. Finally, Berry, too, was pretty sure it was time to stop working on it. "Okay, let's hear the story again," she ordered.

Joe's Mom

My new friend Joe wants me to meet his family. I'm not sure I should do this. He might take it as a signal about us. Just beginning to feel my independence, I've already had a couple of boyfriends since high school—show offs though, not like Joe. Clever, overly confident guys, not always that nice.

Joe is quiet, tender, and funny. Nevertheless, I feel threatened—maybe because he seems so conventional. I fear getting trapped in a life where I can expect to cook dinner, clean house, and raise kids. After putting him off a couple of times, though, I decide to go home with him to meet his mom, dad, and younger brother, Alan.

Their neat suburban house is on the outskirts of Chicago, not far from where my family lives on the north side. It's a new tri-level with the living area on the ground floor and a large family room half-a-flight down. Inside, I find it uncluttered, with plain comfortable furniture. A small lawn in front and a larger one in back are bordered with colorful flowers that must be zinnias.

Joe's mom, Adele, is tall and soft looking—seemingly somewhat reserved, although her smiling eyes make me feel right at home. I watch her as she listens carefully to everyone's experiences of the day, setting the tone for dinner-time conversation. Within a couple of weeks of going home with Joe after school, it's begun to seem as if I've been drawn into the family, soaking up feeling cared for, yet still reluctant—afraid of being trapped and stifled.

Now, on a late fall afternoon, Joe tells me his mom has ovarian cancer. I wonder if she's had it all along or did they just find out? I ask him if he's sure it's okay with her that he told me. Should I show my sympathy for her or pretend I still don't know? It's all right for you to know, he says.

While Adele's still preparing dinners with plenty of beef and potatoes and crunchy salads, I realize she's taking care of us. Never ruffled, she doesn't seem to be dying.

Right now, she's collecting seeds from her zinnias and asters even though she says she may not be here in the spring to plant them. Her husband and sons squirm when she says that. One day, when she hands the seeds to me, I panic. Is this a sign, approving of Joe and me? Is she asking me to be here next year to plant them? If I accept them, will I be obligated to the relationship with Joe? Full of my worries, I'm unable to say more than a weak thank you, hesitantly slipping them into my purse.

Adele continues to perform her duties in the same cheerful manner she must have cultivated as a nurse, trying to protect her husband, Phil, and their boys from the emotional trauma of losing her. One day, over a sink full of dishes, she tells me she was a birthing nurse. She had seen doctors choose not to stimulate babies born with obvious deformities. It gave her pause, she said, but at that time, working in the hospital, she felt she needed to keep her opinions about the doctors' judgments to herself. Does it strengthen her to keep quiet now about her own illness? Having always been there for others, shouldn't she be sharing some of her burden with the family now?

Joe's dad Phil is a balding man of average height, appearing smaller than Adele because of his angularity. His style of doing simple things, such as buying groceries or picking up the dry cleaning, often includes an abundance of worrying and fussing. His hasty movements remind me of a bird building its nest.

The brothers let me understand that their mom is the artist of the garden. One especially dry year, they tell me, Phil tried to help out by watering her plants. He took great care with a particular plant that amazed everyone by growing to be ten feet high. Adele purposely let him nurture this virile weed. Now, Phil affectionately joins the boys in telling the story as a joke on himself. Adele's practical jokes included last April Fools' Day when her exclamations about an unexpected foot of snow got everyone leaping out of bed and running to the windows well before their alarms went off.

In better times, there must have been even more laughter. I'm guessing that in their marriage, Adele's humor has been a balm for Phil's nerves, and his conscientiousness a tranquilizer for what may have been her own anxieties. Their family life, however, still appears to me distressingly predictable.

Joe looks like his mom—tall and blue-eyed with curly blond hair. He observes that the students at the Art Institute, where we both go to college, have given up trying to fit into the culture around them. Instead, many of the boys are bearded and have long hair and the girls wear foreign looking clothes, determined to show their uniqueness by playing up eccentricity.

Joe says we're like cartoons of ourselves. He takes the edge off the signs of inner conflict just like his mom does. His paintings are oversize depictions of lawn chair webbing. In the small spaces of background, you can see landscape or other hints of a world beyond. His lithographs of ordinary objects such as neckties and sneakers convey a startling juiciness. Is this making fun of the objects in his life his way of rebelling against convention?

I've long stopped eating dinner at home, where the TV

guarantees no conversation. Instead, I go to Joe's almost every evening, trying to be helpful, but maybe Joe's mom needs to do everything herself to feel like she's still essential. Allowed small tasks, I set the table or poke the cauliflower to see if it's cooked. Occasionally, she shares a recipe. Is she wondering whether I'm the one Joe might marry? If so, does she approve?

Over the weeks, dinners become increasingly somber. How could the family continue to be playful when the mother is dying? Adele confides to me that by keeping to the daily schedule with no emotional ups and downs, she feels like their family life can stay intact longer. To myself, I wonder, without the passion of our fears and grief, isn't it also more tedious? I can't seem to help judging what they've chosen.

After dinner, we all hang out watching television. Eventually, the rest of the family leaves the room, allowing Joe and me to lie on the couch and cuddle. It's pretty nice until Joe begins scratching the red itchy rash on the inside of his forearms—a rash his father also has.

Every afternoon at 4:20, we could almost set our clocks by Adele feeling her worst. Though she never utters a word, you can tell she's drenched in pain. She just mutely lies down until she can move again. When the wave passes, she disappears into the bathroom where, Joe says, she's taking more codeine. Dare we ask why she doesn't take it before the pain comes back? Seemingly unwilling to step out from our charade, day after day she continues to take care of herself.

When the initial surgery didn't work, she had opted for no more treatment. She'd seen too much of that, she once told us. It's better to die peacefully than prolong the agony and need even more drugs because of what they've done to you. Every few weeks she has a crisis, each one leaving her weaker than the last.

Now, it's almost winter. Adele, having no energy left for functioning, finally allows Phil to take her to the hospital. Each day, he visits her after work while Joe and I are still in school. I wonder if it would be better for us to be with her.

But then, how long would we need to miss school? Now, on the nights I'm at their house, I help Phil prepare dinner or at least set the table for take-out he's brought home. Today, when we ask how she's feeling, he confides to us that she said she knows she will die in the late afternoon when she invariably feels so bad.

Most evenings, we have dinner as early as we can and then go visit her. Although I've overcome my former dread of her illness and the oppressive odor of the hospital, I must still keep an emotional distance. I'm just the new girlfriend, I tell myself. Maybe I don't really know her well enough to be visiting at what seems so intimate a time. Surely she senses my ambivalence.

Sometimes, when the boys are telling her about their day, I think I see fear in her eyes, knowing she won't be able to share their future. But then, love returns to her expression and, as always, she steers the conversation to the practical. It's as if she doesn't want to remember she's dying, as if the kids don't need to talk about it, as if no one longs to find a way to say good-bye.

Each day's rhythm feels the same, like a long train ride. Although we've seemed to agree not to talk about the destination, nevertheless, we arrive. On a Monday, Adele is dead. In spite of months of preparation, we still experience shock. More strange, is that even though Adele had been in the hospital for the last few weeks, only now does the house suddenly feel empty of her presence.

Only a single day is allowed to pass before the memorial service and burial must take place. It is a cold, blustery, wet autumn day, appropriate for a funeral. The commemoration at the chapel is performed by professionals, and, although the room is filled with mourners, there is little feeling of any personal tributes to her spontaneity or bravery. At Shalom Gardens, black umbrellas, like sails on a ship, angle identically against the wind.

Once home again, it is a relief to be out of the biting rain.

Rabbi Levitsky places the traditional shiva mourning candle on the fireplace mantle and suggests that Phil be the one to light it. As he does, the Rabbi says a blessing and then sits with us to explain that it will burn for seven days. This fist-thick candle was made by pouring wax into a glass cylinder, he says, which keeps it from burning unevenly or more quickly than it's supposed to.

After the Rabbi leaves, Joe and I sit with his dad at the dining room table. We're almost basking in the quiet after the tension of being with other people most of the day. In a couple of hours, visitors will arrive with food and memories to begin sitting shiva—the seven-day period of mourning. Phil is musing about Adele, almost talking to himself. The monotonous sound of his voice is soothing, despite its sadness.

"She told me she was sure she was going to die in the late afternoon when she always felt so bad—and she did."

Suddenly, Alan yells from the living room, "Dad, the candle's gone out!" What makes Joe, his father, and me all look in the opposite direction through the kitchen doorway to the clock on the wall?

4:20.

The hair on my arms stands up. Then, I am filled with a sense of reassurance. The house feels almost joyous. Do they sense it, too? We sit a moment, dazed, but then rouse ourselves to rush off and join Alan in the living room where Phil easily relights the candle.

-end-

"No," says Berry. "Wrong word. Say 'where Phil *solemnly* relights the candle.' Read the last paragraph again."

I read it replacing the one word. "How do you do that?" I asked. "It suggests *easily* but conveys the mood we think we ought to be feeling."

Another Day

*For all that ye may ever keep is just what you give away, and
that you give away is advice, counsel, manner of life you live
yourself. The manner in which you treat your fellow man, your
patience, your brotherly love, your kindness, your gentleness.
That you give away, that is all that ye may possess
in those other realms of consciousness.*
- EDGAR CAYCE READING 5259-1

Berry had a request. She'd talked around the topic a number of
times but now she was being direct. "Can you imagine? They want
to charge $40 to give me a pedicure! I have a nail clipper. Would
you cut my nails?"

Admittedly, I had avoided offering her help when she brought
up the subject before. Berry was happy enough to spend $40 on
hummus; why not on her own grooming? You'd think this would
be part of basic care at the home. Why hadn't Kathryn done it?
Then, I reminded myself how dangerous it could be to make a
wound on a foot with so little circulation. My uncle Maury, dia-
betic, took months to heal from a little mistake his doctor had
made. My inner chatter made it apparent I was feeling quite guilty
about not wanting to do it.

Also, could I hide my repugnance? Berry's yellowish nails
looked like hooves, thick, curved, because they hadn't been cut in
so long. I wasn't sure the clippers would even go through them.
Berry must have seen me hanging back and suddenly asked if I'd
cut her fingernails instead. "We could work on the toenails another time," she added.

My apprehension made her fingernails seem easy by contrast.
They were healthy looking, beautiful pink ovals. Now, it wasn't
the task that was a challenge, just the physical awkwardness. Berry
had made it clear early on she didn't like being touched. She
refused to be hugged and had warned me against it the first time I
made a gesture. Only occasionally had she allowed angelic Mary
Jane, who introduced us, to touch her lightly. When Mary Jane

95

was giving Berry a Therapeutic Touch treatment, it actually required no touching at all.

Fingernails cut, the next time I came, Berry again asked about cutting her toenails. She wasn't going to drop the subject so I steeled myself to make an attempt, beginning with her baby toe. The clipper might have a chance of being able to cut through it, I thought. Very carefully planting it around the nail, I clipped.

"Ouch! You nipped me."

"Oh, Berry, I can't do this. That's just what I thought I was being so careful to avoid. You've got to get a professional. This isn't my kind of thing." Why hadn't I insisted on that in the first place? I felt so beholden to Berry, I couldn't say, 'No'.

The whole nail trimming incident reminded me of my retreating nature in sharp contrast to the boldness Berry expressed in her childhood story about little Carolyn. When she had told me that story I revealed one of my own obtuse ventures around the same age.

Contrary to Mom's usual remoteness, she had tried in her way to rescue me from a difficulty at school. In second grade, Mrs. Mallov gave us a task to do as soon as we arrived in the morning. Its purpose was to quiet everyone down until the official start of the school day when the bell rang. We were to copy what she had put on the black board—a weather report and a drawing of a thermometer indicating the temperature. I was painstakingly careful in my work, yet sending myself off to school in the morning always resulted in arriving at what was theoretically considered on time— moments before the bell. Therefore, I could never finish the assignment before it was collected. Each day before lunch my paper would be returned to me and instead of receiving a beautiful gold star there was always an ugly turkey stamped on it in red ink!

Our house was only a block from school so I always walked home for lunch with an unconscious feeling of growing frustration from this daily disapproval. One afternoon I refused to go back to school. My stomach hurt, I told my mother. She didn't let me stay home, however. She would go back with me, she said, and talk to the teacher. Mom asked Mrs. Mallov if I was a good student.

"Oh, yes!"

"Does she behave herself?"

"I never have any trouble with her," the teacher answered.

"Is her printing good?" Mom asked.

"Exceptional. Very neat and legible."

"But every day you give her a turkey..."

My mother had reminded me of this story shortly before she died, proud of having arranged with Mrs. Mallov that I would be a 'helper' in class in order to receive a little positive attention from her. She *did* understand I was unhappy but why hadn't she and the teacher addressed the possibility of my coming to school a few minutes earlier to deal directly with the symbol of daily failure—the dreaded red turkey?

Berry was struggling with her little sausage shaped pillow again. "Put that under my shoulders, would you? You confirm in my mind that there were certain benefits to not going to school."

I said, "I'm sure if I hadn't been allowed, that would have been the only thing I'd have wanted." Then getting back to the subject of teachers, I said, "I had thought Mrs. Mallov was demanding, but in fourth grade, Mrs. Widener was even more threatening. She told us that she had been an actress. A piece of her personal history she let us know was that she had broken her right arm—the hand she wrote with.

"'It was simple', she told us, 'I learned to write with my other hand.' Her intent might have been to inspire us with what can be accomplished when needed. Instead, it affirmed in my mind that we didn't have a chance in hell against her superior powers."

Berry laughed and then was quiet while her trembling hands made a rasping sound, fingers rubbing against the sheets. This time it seemed exceptionally loud to me.

"Each day," I said, "some incident would lend itself to a drama that would underscore Mrs. Widener's control of us. A boy accused of stealing change from another child, for instance, was put on trial. She had another student take down the classroom flag and hold it in front for him swear on.

"In a booming voice, with threats of what might happen to him if he were to lie, she asked, 'Do you swear to tell the truth, the whole truth, and nothing but the truth?' The accused broke out in a sweat. All of us in the room were shaking in commiseration. Did we find him guilty? I have no memory of that—only the high drama of intensifying fear.

"Another day, she made a very self-conscious person in class— an unusually tall girl with kinky red hair—sing by herself in front of us. You could practically hear her knees knocking. Each day presented a new humiliation. Never had it seemed more important to be invisible. Every night, in bed I would cry myself to sleep, fearful of what might happen the following day. My parents never asked what I was crying about."

Berry's hands went still, "How could they be so unfeeling?"

"I never understood. By this time, I was deep into a precocious bedtime eroticism, begun, perhaps, because of so many sleepless nights. It was the only thing that would put me to sleep. That, they were preternaturally aware of. They would yell from their room, 'Go to sleep!' I must have been doing something really bad."

How I Seemed

If you want to build a ship,
don't herd people together to collect wood and
don't assign them tasks and work, but rather
teach them to long for the endless immensity of the sea.
- ANTOINE DE SAINT-EXUPERY

Berry's receptiveness drew my words out, allowing them to take form, like a flourishing plant. I'd often be as surprised as she over some of the things I said to her.

On a day when we'd been conjecturing about how different cultures viewed psychology, I described a shamanic viewpoint, the shaman being a healing person.

"When we experience a traumatic event," I said, "the part of our soul that is unable to deal with it leaves and lives in another reality. Missing pieces make it harder to respond well to new challenges here. In order to function fully, we need those sensitivities that have gone into hiding. Bringing those pieces back is what they call soul retrieval."

"It makes so much sense!" Berry exclaimed. "They found a way to restore our wholeness."

"Those cultures make no differentiation between health and spirituality," I said. "In our culture we think everything is separate from spirit instead of everything being related to it."

Berry was practically smacking her lips, "Exactly!"

There was no stopping me now. "This dichotomy developed when there was a need to separate learning from the politics of the Church. Now we've carried this notion to such an extreme that people have lost contact with the ephemeral world of qualities. We're fundamentalist materialists." I sounded like I knew what I was talking about. But my intensity should have been a clue I still hadn't really integrated that understanding.

Eyes sparkling, Berry revealed an experience that had unbalanced her. "When that ephemeral world broke through to me," she said, "I didn't know how to relate to it. I had no trouble in sep-

99

arating my inner life from the outer world until I was about sixteen. But suddenly, I found myself in the middle of a war of words—poetry mixed in with the Dow Jones average. 'When in disgrace with fortune in men's eyes, I all alone bewail my outcast state since volume declined on this heavy selling...' I actually couldn't talk. It was the worst suffering I'd ever experienced. Fortunately, I was still able to take dictation at work. Only after much prayer did my confusion lift." Then Berry seemed to gaze into a dark distance, unseen by me. "Not until I discovered the balm of alcohol at about eighteen, could I bear to remember this awful strife."

We looked into each others' eyes.

"I've never experienced anything like that," I said, finally remembering to take a deep gratifying breath. "My conflicts were...are quieter. Often, I'm barely able to articulate anything about that inner world. It's a feeling that something is there, like a dream I know I had but can't remember. It makes me chronically uncomfortable, but ultimately the outer world, the one we agree about, is always so much louder, always overshadowing everything else."

A burst of laughter from the hall broke our mood—nurses joking as they walked past the room.

Suddenly I asked, "Did I tell you about the spoon-bending party I arranged a few months before I met you?

"Spoon-bending? Berry repeated.

"I met the man at a conference a couple of years ago, when I was writing the *Healing Arts Report*. I accidently found out about the conference on the Internet. The sponsoring organization's acronym ISSSEEM stands for the International Society for the Study of Subtle Energies and Energy Medicine. The acronym read as 'I seem' made me think they, at least, had a sense of humor so I looked around the site and discovered it had been founded by a well-known scientist, Elmer Green. I remembered hearing about Elmer and Alyce Green in the '60s. They were husband and wife, renowned for their research in the field of biofeedback, measuring brain waves and correlating them with meditative states and the ability to effect change in what until then had been considered involuntary bodily processes."

Loud pounding from out in the hall was repeatedly drowning out my voice. "What are they doing—remodeling?" I asked Berry.

"They're breaking pills."

I laughed at what I thought was her absurd joke and was soundly rebuked.

"They do this every day, at least twice a day," Berry insisted.

Unbelieving, I got up and peeked down the hall, still sure, because of the loudness, I was going to see several carpenters with tools and a ladder. Instead, it was exactly as Berry said, two nurses hovering over a medicine cart, one looking at notes on her clipboard and the other smashing down a little silver lever on a contraption small enough to be hidden by her hand. When I walked down the hall to them and asked what was going on, the nurse answered that she was breaking pills.

"How in the world could it make that much noise?"

Barely looking up, with a little shrug of her shoulders, she said, "That's how it works."

"We can't even hear ourselves talk," I said, pointing to Berry's room.

"I guess you'd better close the door."

I stomped back to the room shaking my head. "Who invented that? And why would a nursing home choose to use it?" I said, indulging my annoyance.

"I've got to write a story about a nursing home!" Berry said laughing. "There's so much humorous material here. After I finish the memoirs, we'll do it. Of course," she added, "we'll have to keep it a secret from the authorities."

Laughing, again, we took deep breaths in tandem and then Berry prompted, "You were telling me about a conference."

"Oh yes. ISSSEEM was to have a conference in Boulder. When I got there, I was pleased to find the participants as engaging a collection of people as I'd hoped for. They described themselves as mystics who were interested in science and scientists who considered themselves mystics."

I explained that Bill Gough, the chairman of the conference, was a retired nuclear engineer with a lifetime of experience in the world of science. He said that as he came across mysteries that couldn't be explained by conventional models, he began searching for an expanded scientific paradigm. This conference was almost a forum for his explorations. He had followed the work and personally knew most of the presenters.

Berry's look of bright interest encouraged me to keep talking.

"One night, it was announced there was going to be an event that wasn't on the schedule—a spoon-bending party! Do you remember Uri Geller, the Israeli psychokinetic entertainer who was supposed to be bending spoons with the power of his mind?"

"Oh, yes, there was a lot of hype," Berry said. "He bent keys and watch hands, too. They'd show him on TV, forehead dripping with the efforts of concentration."

"Frankly, I never understood what all the fuss was about. Most likely it was a trick, but even if it weren't, why would you want to bend spoons?

"Now, in the context of healing, I finally realized the implications. My disregard suddenly seemed so foolish. A person's beliefs define her life. Yet, somehow the idea of being able to manipulate the material world with the mind is more convincing about its power. Isn't that silly?" I asked.

Berry answered thoughtfully, "We think whatever we believe is true—and we believe the material world is the one that counts."

At the convention I became giddy from meeting so many people interested in the subjects we were studying. It seemed like a spoon-bending party would be just that much *more* fun so I signed up. Everyone else must have been feeling that way, too. There was a buzz of expectation as we arrived and seated ourselves. About seventy-five people gathered in the red carpeted conference room, waiting for Jack Houck to arrive. Unlike the other hotel meeting rooms, this ground-level one had a low ceiling which created a feeling of intimacy. We moved our folding chairs into informal concentric circles with a space in the middle for Jack to make his presentation.

Berry asked me if I had known who he was. I only knew what I'd been told there—that he was an aeronautical engineer, a defense consultant about 'Star Wars' technology for the government. They said he'd had a TV show in California about the power of the mind. Later, I read a short reference about him in Jim Schnabel's book *Remote Viewers: The Secret History of America's Psychic Spies*. I didn't know what I'd been expecting, but when he finally entered the room, I was amused to see a compact little man looking like the quintessential accountant. He wore a suit with a white shirt and necktie, and was hefting a huge suitcase.

The room became quiet as he greeted us, stepping into the circle. Then he opened the latch, noisily spilling out hundreds of spoons and forks, setting off our laughter. Later, at the time of our bending experiment, he showed us some square aluminum rods about three feet long. When he placed them, one end on the floor and the other on a chair seat, we couldn't bend them even by jumping on them.

Jack spent well over an hour telling us about his background, how he first heard of spoon-bending from a friend at work. Being a scientist, he cut utensils that had been bent in order to examine their molecular structure. He drew diagrams on the blackboard, all the while making us laugh—at him, science, the government, ourselves, even psychokinesis. This lecture went on for so long, I considered the possibility that he was hypnotizing us. Not to make us see things that weren't there, but just using the time to break down our preconceptions, like when you go to a different country and begin to assimilate the expectations of that culture. I could almost sense my own beliefs slowly loosening their grip.

Jack told us about the first spoon-bending party he had ever organized. "I invited the neighbors," he said, "encouraging them to bring their children. Kids are very good at this," he pointed out, "because they don't have the biases we adults have."

In preparation for the event, he had pulled out his grandmother's silver, not really expecting anything to happen and showed everyone the technique that his friend had shown him. Much to his own surprise, everyone succeeded except one lady. He explained to us, "She felt that it was a shame to ruin perfectly good silverware. So, of course, she didn't." He also said his mother had never forgiven him for the damage done to most of it.

When I paused, Berry smiled and moved to prop herself up on her right elbow. I lamented about the power of our beliefs. Hadn't I seen this phenomenon in action dozens of times? In art classes you'd hear, "Oh, I can't even draw a straight line!" as if someone couldn't be taught to run a pencil alongside a ruler! Or, "I can't eat that" about food the person had never even tasted. Dozens of beliefs about not being able to do something when all we need is the intention, a little information, and, then, experience.

Somehow I'd given little thought to applying this challenge to things *I* didn't believe were possible. Actually, I thought I believed in all possibilities—only not for me, personally. At this event, I finally realized this might apply to *my* beliefs, too. Bending the flatware that evening didn't even matter any more. What in life, I asked myself, might I want to do that hadn't before seemed possible?

The tension built as we wondered if he were ever going to begin doing it. His long talk was escalating our eagerness. Finally, Jack showed us the process in steps, starting with what he called the kindergarten level. At this stage you used your hands to do the bending. But we prepared in the same way we would later when using only the mind. Step one: Imagine a mass of energy above your head, connect with it, pulling it down through the head, neck, arm, and hand into the utensil. Two: Scream, "Bend! Bend! Bend!" Three: Purposely let go mentally, turning your attention to something else. Then return your attention and bend the utensil.

I remembered reading about this same pattern in scientific research on sending psychic messages. It's the same situation many of us have experienced when finding ourselves thinking intensely about someone. We let go of the thought by getting back to whatever business was at hand, and then the person phones. "Isn't that funny," we tell them, "I was just thinking of you!"

When we used our hands to bend the flatware, we were to twist the handle around at least three times. Many of us agreed that it felt as if we were using less than our full physical strength and the sensation of bending the metal had almost a gooey quality which would stop suddenly and you could no longer bend it.

When it came time to try, we were all doing it at the same time, laughing and screaming, distracting each other and amazing ourselves. We looked—and felt—like inmates of a madhouse. I told all this to Berry.

She remained silent, smiling, with her eyes locked on mine.

Then I added, "There was a hierarchy of difficulty in the flatware Jack brought: Pressed light weight stainless was the easiest, then cast stainless, then silver-plated metal. Some people worked their way up to bending the bowl of a spoon. For the mind-only bend, Jack had us use the light-weight pressed stuff. The handle or a tine bent forward or back just a little for some of us, including myself, and folded completely over for others, but at least two people there were able to bend the square aluminum rods."

I didn't even get around to telling Berry about our local event until the next visit.

Spoon-Bending In Virginia

Some day after we have mastered the winds,
the waves and gravity,
we will harness for God the energies of love;
and then for a second time in the history of the world,
humans will have discovered fire.

- TEILHARD DE CHARDIN

I had pulled my chair into place and sat down facing Berry, who looked well-rested. After our greetings, she reminded me about the spoon-bending story. Again, she knew exactly where we'd left off.

"You said you'd arranged an event like the one in Colorado."

I explained how it had come about. "Ever since last summer when I planned to take a hypnosis course in the fall, I wanted to contact Jack to see if he would come out here. I looked forward to the laughter as much as anything. He said he'd do it for free, if I'd just cover his expenses—the flight from California and an overnight stay. The Healing Arts Council politely passed on my suggestion of our sponsoring him so I was on my own."

"You mean you had a spoon-bending party right around here?" Berry asked, as she struggled to adjust her pillow, again.

I stood up to help push it under her back. "Well, in Winchester. And we held it in the Medical Center Conference room. I thought the venue added a little authority to the scene." Berry smiled. "I ran an ad with Jack's picture in the paper, hawked it to my fellow employees at FEMA and even got my niece and Bruce to come. I loved being able to share part of my real life with my niece who lives so far away. She seemed to enjoy the Auntie Mame-like adventure. And Bruce was a good host—helping organize, taking registrations, making people feel comfortable when they first arrived.

"Jack walked us through the same exercises as he had in Boulder but it was particularly gratifying and nerve-wracking to have so many people there whom I knew personally. Gratifying to be able to share some part of myself I usually hide and nerve-wracking because I was so invested in wanting them to have a good time. No one bent the square rods as far as I know but a few spoon bowls had been crushed. Jack took a video tape of the participants marching past him smiling into the camera and holding up their twisted utensils. He mailed them still shots of themselves. It was great fun, though not so dramatic as the event in Boulder, maybe just because I was too worried about coordinating it. But everyone here seemed to me to be a little more doubting.

"Even preparing for the event had been exciting. To save Jack the difficulty of bringing all the flatware, I supplied the preliminary stuff. He said he'd bring the light weight stuff we could more easily bend with our minds. At Goodwill, finding only a few stray forks and spoons, I almost panicked. Hunting down an employee,

I asked desperately if they had anything in back. He led me first to another employee who then escorted me to a spacious sunlit store room. She pointed to a huge box filled with flatware that must have taken months for them to accumulate. I bought hundreds of utensils for only forty dollars.

"I left behind all the knives. They probably thought I was supplying a reformatory dining hall. You know, there was a strange thing that happened before Jack arrived. Suddenly, I had become uncomfortable about the accommodations I'd arranged for him and his wife in a beautiful colonial-style bed and breakfast just around the corner from my house. The discomfort became so intense that, without knowing why, I canceled the reservation a week before he was to come and paid for other accommodations five miles away.

"When I saw Jack up close in my own home, I realized he was older than I thought and that he seemed to be suffering from arthritis. It took some effort for him to get up to our second story living room. It was then when I understood what was wrong with the original bed and breakfast. The room they were to be in had a colonial style bed requiring a three-step stool to get up into it and the 'in-room' bath had six stairs going down to it."

Shaman

...the big news shamanism offers is not
that the head is connected to the rest of the body,
but that we are not alone.
- MICHAEL HARNER

I was still drifting into reciting to myself the litany of recent wounds: twelve hundred dollars on car repair, car totalled, the police report blaming me for being rear-ended, the death of sweet Gracie whom I'd tamed 14 years before, and, finally, being told the new job wasn't a good fit. How was I going to pull myself out of this funk, nevermind being 59 years old and still feeling as if I hadn't found my place in the world? With all of these affronts so close together, despondence prevailed in spite of my invigorating time with Berry.

I found a little peace in meditation when able to attune beyond my daily drama. Small inklings gave a ripening sense that something was again, as in the sixties, afoot in the world. Writing with Berry inspired me to look back to notes in my journal. From a conference, I had jotted down a few comments from a talk by anthropologist, Alberto Villardo.

"In science," he had said, "if the hypothesis doesn't work, throw it out. In religion, if the hypothesis doesn't work, throw out the facts. In shamanism, follow your own footsteps.

"Shamanism isn't a religion, but it is the basis of all religion.

"Inka elders believe we've come to the end of our species and a new species is being born right now—homo luminous."

These ideas reminded me of Damian, a shaman I had in mind the previous year to do a workshop for the Healing Arts Council. The Council hadn't wanted to sponsor him. Too radical, I guess, for staying in the good graces of the local medical establishment. That's how I'd come to thinking about asking him for a personal soul retrieval.

When I phoned, he said, "Just asking for this indicates a commitment to change." Encouraged, I felt a cheerful anticipation to working in a way that I hoped would be more natural to me. The appointment was set for the week Bruce was to be at his employer's annual meeting. It seemed a good thing to have no requirements from home, just have the experience and take time to digest it.

A few days before the appointment, however, I began to get anxious, first, over having to drive into the city through the streaming traffic, then, from it being a holiday weekend. Won't the roads be even more crowded than usual? Always troubled by finding my way to new places, I wondered if I'd be able to follow his directions. Would people be riding my tail while I was trying to read street signs? I took a number of precautions to quiet my busy mind: I wrote out the directions in large print with a black marker so I could see them while driving. I filled the gas tank, checked the oil, and last, charged the cell phone battery, as if these things would address the real cause of my insecurity.

When it was time to leave, I thought, I don't even know Damian. Maybe he lives in a dangerous neighborhood. Had I heard a dangerous edge to his voice? What if he's a big scary-looking guy? I left a note on my dining room table with all the appointment information, his address and phone number. I was going to his home, for godssake! Why didn't I find out more?

It had been enough for me that someone I knew took a workshop from him, but suddenly that didn't seem like enough. I got his name over the Internet. How foolish!... well, actually from a respected authority and author about shamanism I'd known of for over twenty years, a world renowned anthropologist. But I didn't know him either. Oh, honestly, and Damian had been around for years at the same phone number, listed with the organization. And then it began to pour. I hated driving in the rain. Finally finding one positive angle, I said to myself, Thank goodness, it's daylight.

The directions were impeccable. With ten minutes to spare, I turned off the engine and sat awhile, breathing and enjoying the rhythmic sound of rain drops on the car roof. I could see the entrance to Damian's house from where I'd parked. Then it was time to knock on the door.

When he opened it, I looked into the face of a regular person, just a few inches taller than I. I felt comfortable immediately. He suggested I take my shoes off and sit where I liked in the living room. Set up with cushions on the floor, there were also chairs for those who preferred them. The rug was Native American. Drums, stacks of CDs, a stereo, nothing jarring about the surroundings. He gently invited me to share a little more background about my concerns.

After I did, he explained what the session would consist of. I would be lying down as he shook a rattle. Then he would sit next to me in contact with my shoulder.

"Some shamans lie down next to the person, but I would fall asleep," he explained laughing. "Usually, I search for three soul pieces and will bring them back to you, blowing them into your solar plexus while you are still lying down and again into the crown of your head after I help you sit up. We will talk about what I've done and then you will lie down again to integrate them while I play chimes and a brass bowl for about five minutes. When you hear a whistle, that indicates the ceremony is finished."

I lay down and closed my eyes as Damian began. Immediately I had a vision of my own.

I am surrounded by aborigines I recognize from a vision years before. I am lying next to a camp fire which they are sitting around. Also here to help me are Grandpa Israel's grandmother whom I call Laughing Lady, the ancient oriental gentleman who gives blessings, Granny D., and Jim, a dead friend. Oryx is here, too, licking the baby oryx.

She says to me, "This is normal. All babies deserve this just because they exist. They don't have to earn it. It is available from the universe. If someone is kind to you, you don't owe them a piece of your soul in exchange. Kindness is what the universe expects from us. Don't ever sell yourself short to anyone just because they treat you decently. Decent treatment is what you have the right to expect."

One of the aborigines tells me they aren't going to do anything but be with me. Granny D.'s presence without having asked for her is a gift. I chuckle as the old oriental gentleman reminds me to half smile (a technique that always makes me laugh). He says, "You'll be able to breathe easier," which is exactly what happens. I feel grateful that they're here to be with me.

Comforted by Damian's contact against my shoulder, I waited for him to return from his vision. When he was finished blowing the parts back into my solar plexus and head, he told me what he found.

"Maybe I wouldn't have found the infant if you had not told me of your worry about her. When I picked her up and cuddled her, your parents suddenly showed up, distressed. 'What are you doing?' they wanted to know. I reassured them that you'd be all right. I explained I was taking you to be with their now grown-up daughter. They seemed to accept that."

"That's just like them," I said, "to be all worried when someone shows up, yet they hadn't been with me themselves."

Damian continued without responding to my flash of anger, "I next met a college co-ed BJ. She was a fire brand, gone off because college was so ordinary. She was ready to revolutionize the world. Vital, active, hoping to make a mark on the planet."

Yes, I thought, I had been so disappointed to see what the students at art school were like. I had expected to learn from them how to change the world but they were intent on looking for a path to success in the conventional sense—gallery representation, getting their art into museums.

Damian described still more. "Then, I visited a future you, about 75 years old. I found her beautiful, graceful, vital. She sent a message to you, 'You have nothing to lose.' Then, she became around 35-years-old, filled with energy, ready for action, and she added, 'Believe in yourself and in the help that surrounds you.'"

You'd think I already would. After all, didn't I identify all those helpers around the campfire? How is it that as soon as they're out of sight, I forget about them?

Lost in thought, I suddenly became aware again of Damian sitting in front of me, bringing my attention back to what he was saying. "I often make it a point to see the oversoul, or BJ Central, as I like to call it. I was told that you need to acquire personal power. If there is a theme to this session, it is the regaining of lost vitality."

Apparently, not one to assume anything, he asked me, "Are these images relevant; do they make sense?"

"They all make sense," I answered, but I didn't tell him that the suggestion to acquire personal power caused a sudden surge of inner whining. I immediately started saying to myself, 'I can't *do* that. I don't know how.'

During the integration time, when I lay down again, my collegiate self started talking to me.

"I left," she said, "when you got mononucleosis. seeing how frightened you were to be living away from home and how needy you were for companionship. You were willing to accept such poor expressions of so-called love. I was disgusted."

"Well, maybe I wouldn't have been so fearful and needy if you hadn't left," I said defensively.

"Instead of doing something out in the world," she countered, "you spent all your time looking for love."

"Maybe I needed love in order to feel secure enough to do things out in the world," I said, continuing to justify myself even after realizing she had been frightened by my behavior.

She reiterated, "I hated seeing you so vulnerable, and then, after your illness, so weak physically. It was more than I could bear. You put yourself—us—in danger by seeking love all the time.

I knew she was right and got a hold of myself. "I'm sorry to have scared you. I need you now. Without you, I'm not fully alive. Also," I asked, suddenly curious, "are you able to do things in this world without me?"

No, she couldn't.

I became pensive, "I was repulsed by me, too. Without vitality, that hungry person seemed to be all that I was." Then, taking a breath, I said, "I didn't mean to blame you. I've often thought about how that state I was in fostered risk. Now, we could help each other..."

Damian's voice intruded. "You'll continue to work on integration at home," he said. "Let me know what you've done."

With the session completed, he invited me to the kitchen for a drink of water or juice. Feeling a little shaky, I was glad to accept the sweet pineapple juice. He said casually, "Maybe you know my sister, Lena. She lives in Berryville near where you live." My brain began tumbling like an old fashioned slot machine. The first row spinning names and stopping at their shared last name. The second row matching the name with the town. Bells went off!

"Why, I've known her for 25 years! We were on a dance team together." As I quieted myself and looked directly at him, it was easy to see the family resemblance. Inside, I couldn't help laughing at myself, contrasting my earlier anxiety with the feeling now, standing in the kitchen with him, of his seeming more like a long lost relative.

Though he appeared as shy as I, as I stepped out the door, he leaned forward in a subtle gesture to give me a hug and I was happy for the fleeting embrace.

Reality

I am always doing that which I cannot do,
in order that I may learn how to do it.
- PABLO PICASSO (1881 - 1973)

I told Berry about the shamanic session with Damian after the fact.

She said, "I'm glad I didn't know about it beforehand. The trouble with thinking of you as another daughter is that I'm beginning to worry about you, too."

I squeezed Berry's hand. "I had told Damian how I was always trying to find balance in my life and, how, in the end, I never pleased the people around me nor myself. You should have seen his reaction. He sneered!

"'Who says balance is so great? Doing things by half-measure is what I call it. Humph! A misguided notion.'

"I thought about what he said. I had to admit that whenever I heard people talking about their success with something, it was just the opposite of what I'd always done. They filled their life with it. They became fanatics, devoted to the thing they loved doing, against all reason!"

"Isn't that what I've been saying? You should just write."

I didn't respond to Berry's gentle chide, because I still couldn't see how I could do that. I wasn't even sure I wanted to do that. Instead I said, "I also told him how 'altered reality' experiences I've had have been the most real experiences of my life, changing me, yet something in me wants, like the rest of the culture, to doubt them.

"Damian said casually, 'That's normal. When I catch myself doing that I just tell my brain, You can go there if you want but I'll just continue about my business. Don't worry about it. Don't argue with it. Just let it do its thing.'"

Berry and I sat quietly, the only sound, her vibrating hands rubbing against the sheet.

Leaving Home

There is a very simple reason why we have a sense of insecurity, because we do not agree to be what we are.
- J.G. BENNETT

Berry was well into the second section of her memoirs, still talking about her childhood. This story must have been from during the Depression. She said that due to the collapse of the economy, her mother had to return from Colorado with Berry and her little brother Darrell who had eventually joined them out west. They were again living with the grandparents, the children having their first school experience, enforced by their grandfather. It wasn't more than a month after their return to Mississippi that their beloved Grandmama died.

Without her modulating influence, the antagonism between Berry's mother and grandfather quickly escalated, becoming insufferable. He accused his daughter of malingering and demanded she take on the duties of her mother and their longtime maid, whom he fired. Quickly exhausted by the work, she came up with a plan.

She took her children by stealth to Louisiana where the first thing she did was purchase a bicycle for Darrell who took a job selling newspapers. With Berry, she began perusing the want ads to find her a job. She was 15. After days of fruitless inquiry, Berry had an idea inspired by familiarity with her grandfather's bank, to go into one and ask for work. She described wandering around the intimidating lobby looking for someone to speak to until finally a man came over to her.

"He asked if he could help me. I told him how our family had a bank and that I wondered if I could work here. He invited me to sit at his polished mahogany desk while he went to get an older gentleman from one of the wainscotted offices. I let them believe I was my ill mother's sole support."

Berry referred to these men as her fairy godfathers because, without her having any qualifications, they gave her the opportunity to prove she could do the job.

"I left with application in hand, running home to the sound of deafening applause." My laughter didn't slow Berry down. She smiled beatifically. "My mother could hardly believe our good fortune and made immediate plans for me to learn shorthand before the starting date. She would test me by having me transcribe an article she read from the newspaper each day.

"When Darrell came home, he was immediately dispatched with an alarming number of dollar bills to purchase a celebratory feast from the Syrian store." Then she paused. "Let's make that a Jewish delicatessen. What are some Jewish foods?"

Eager to participate in her story, I began listing them. "Corned beef, lox, cream cheese, smoked fish, gefilte fish, onion rolls, bialys, kosher pickles..."

"And what kind of dessert?"

"Very plain cake, no frosting, like a sponge cake."

"Sponge cake," she reiterated.

Perhaps Berry had been imagining that my interest was flagging. She knew the food of my childhood, mostly unknown around here, would get my attention. To her, if the deli story weren't true in fact, it was in spirit.

"To a writer," she stressed, "that's all that counts."

Downtown, doing some errands, I met my friend Georgia by chance. I remembered that she was one of the people that had lived with Berry on her farm. She already knew about Berry's illness and had even visited when Berry first entered the nursing home.

"In the middle of a conversation," Georgia explained, "Berry suddenly just stared up at the ceiling. Thinking she might be having a stroke, I said to her, 'Berry, are you all right? It's me, Georgia, do you know who I am?.' Berry became incensed and chased me away."

I knew the look Georgia described and sympathized with her reaction. I saw it a lot when Berry was thinking. Her eyes would roll up to the ceiling and she'd go perfectly still for a long while. Even her tremors would stop. Probably only my chronic timidity had saved me from doing the same thing Georgia had done.

When I next saw Berry, I conveyed greetings to her from Georgia. Berry launched into a description of the same visit, adding, "Imagine her asking if I knew her. I'm sick, for godssake, not senile!"

The Culture As Health

... thank you thank you thank you for the breathtaking mystery
of us all here together in the crucible of time
working out our salvation with diligence.

- ROB BREZSNY

As soon as I was seated, Berry said, "What I really have a taste for now is sauerkraut."

I wrinkled up my nose. "You love that sour taste, don't you? You also like the sourest flavors of hummus."

"I could drink vinegar," she said. "But I don't think they have live sauerkraut anymore, just the canned stuff that's been cooked."

"Well, you'll be glad to know that the grocery does have the real thing—packaged in cellophane. They sell it in the meat department."

"Would you bring some next time?" she asked. "And if you could run it through a blender for a couple of minutes, that would make it a lot easier for me to eat."

I relished getting Berry something she craved. There wasn't too much left in the material world she cared about. Little gifts people brought were immediately abandoned to collecting dust on the window sill. What could she do with them? I wrote myself a reminder and turned off the sound from the ever-droning TV. The sudden quiet, always an instant balm, made me take a deep breath.

"I'm going to teach some free classes," I announced. "I've picked dates for giving one at the local library and several more at the Center in Winchester. The newspaper will list freebies. At the classes, I'll promote longer workshops that have a fee. That way I won't have to buy expensive ads. I'll also make some flyers to leave at the health food stores."

Always alert to another one of my schemes, Berry asked, "What's the first class about?"

"It'll be an overview. I'm calling it *What's All The Fuss About Alternative Medicine?*"

Smiling, she said, "You better read it to me."

I loved Berry's tone of motherly concern, but I hadn't intended to write my lecture. "I just use an outline that I'll talk from."

"Well, you need to give the talk to me. I can play devil's advocate and let you know whether you're getting your points across."

That *would* be helpful, I thought. Berry was interested in alternative medicine but she seemed to understand it the way most people did—as a natural substitute for drugs—not really a different concept.

"I'll bring my notes," I said with conviction. Then I plugged in the laptop and inserted a disk. Berry tsked over my having to fuss with the broken hinges as I gingerly opened it.

"When we sell a story, we'll get you a new computer," she said.

"That would really be great!" I answered as I was thinking, Let's hope it holds up while Berry is still writing.

She said, "Read what I wrote from the beginning of the second section."

As we worked on it we talked about some of the incidents. Her grandfather had returned from a trip to Vicksberg late at night and when she heard him groaning the next morning, in her mind, she had him dead and buried, the path cleared for her to take over.

"I imagined myself without tears yet sorrowful, supervising the funeral. My pleasant thoughts were cut short when, a few minutes later, I could hear my grandparents talking about escaped calves and a late milkman."

Berry was great at painting a portrait of herself as a child tyrant. After a couple more pages, she was through dictating for the day and we resumed our discussion.

I got on a soapbox contending that doctors should be exemplary—role models for health—just as professors were supposed to have expertise in the subjects they taught.

"We've put doctors on such a high pedestal they aren't even under common sense scrutiny. Why would anyone trust a 300-pound doctor to help them lose weight? Isn't it obvious there's something he doesn't understand?" I ranted, much to Berry's delight.

Preparing For The Third Story

Creativity is not the finding of a thing,
but the making something out of it after it is found.
- JAMES RUSSELL LOWELL (1819-1891)

Every now and then something new would appear on the wall next to Berry's window. This time it was a child's drawing, perhaps a self-portrait, taped next to photos of all the grandchildren. Berry occasionally mentioned them to me. A vase of flowers that had materialized on the window sill weeks before, I noticed, was now completely shrivelled, tended to by neither visitors nor staff.

I arrived that day with the beginning of my next story, which Berry set me to read. It took place years ago when I went to Crete. Before it was barely begun, she had me remove descriptions of my fellow travellers—a couple of actors from Chicago, blond California hikers, a woman travelling alone. "They delay our getting into the story," she explained. I couldn't quite recognize it. The people I was with *were* the story, weren't they? But, Berry had a seasoned way of discriminating what was relevant.

After removing the offending material, I began to get an inkling for what she meant. Diversions into description when one was looking for action didn't work. The same thing often happened in my life, I realized.

"You know," I admitted to her, "because of my issues with memory, I'm always so amazed by being able to dredge up anything that I feel compelled to include it. Each tidbit, each interaction seems so precious, I have no discrimination as to its value in the story."

"You will. Your devotion to details may serve to keep the story based in reality but not every aspect has equal weight."

Each visit I'd bring in as much as I had written and Berry would have me read it to her, usually starting from the very beginning, then including the new material. I'd already have gone over each addition a dozen times at home but reading it aloud made me notice things that reading to myself had not. And, of course, Berry

119

always had her suggestions.

Over a period of weeks, alternating with her own writing, Berry listened to the story again and again.

"Don't you get bored?" I asked.

"Never, do you?"

"Well, no, but it's my story. I can work a sentence over for hours."

"My editor," Berry said with a tinge of pride, "used to tell me I was a better editor than a writer. What amazes me is how hard you're willing to work. This is such a pleasure for me. It makes you a great student. I love doing this."

Her enthusiasm pleased me. "The process of writing is fascinating," I said, "I feel fortunate that you're willing to spend so much time on these stories with me. It's like having a private course."

These appreciations, which we had fairly often, always caused me to sing in my head, 'We be-long to a mu-tu-al-l-l-l ad-mir-a-tion so-ci-et-y, my Berry and me.'

After we'd worked on the story for about three weeks, Berry decided something was missing at the very beginning. Maybe that's why she had kept having me read from the start each time.

"There needs to be some kind of introduction," she explained, "something that states the direction—if not a question, some sense that the story has a destination."

To find out what that might be, she asked me about the archaeology of Crete. Berry thought what I told her was interesting and relevant enough to include some of it. The introduction turned into three short paragraphs. For me, her questions expanded my understanding of why the experience still carried some unresolved intensity. What had originally been yet another tale about unexplained misgivings became reflections of a larger drama, a greater perspective.

As usual, upon arriving at the nursing home next visit, I greeted Berry, adjusted the blinds, moved the breakfast tray to the sink, and checked on how she wanted the angle of the bed. Then I announced we could go through the whole story. After about six weeks I'd finally finished it. She said, "Okay, read."

I opened my manila folder while she settled into a new position adjusting the little black sausage pillow. While turning my attention to reading, I caught a glimpse of fresh spots of food decorating her high-necked jersey.

The Third Story—Paradise

Sooner or later we all discover that
the important moments in life are not the advertised ones,
not the birthdays, the graduations, the weddings,
not the great goals achieved.
The real milestones are less prepossessing.
They come to the door of memory unannounced,
stray dogs that amble in, sniff around a bit
and simply never leave.
Our lives are measured by these.
- SUSAN B. ANTHONY (1820-1906)

Paradise

From Athens we had decided to go to Crete, one of the few places in Europe I specifically had a desire to visit. Something about the ancient art drew me.

In the years that have passed since travelling there, I'd begun to wonder why I had never written about it though I'd often spoken to friends about the radiance of the island. Was the overwhelming sadness I felt due to the loss of a beautiful civilization, or was there something malevolent about the culture that I hadn't allowed myself to consider?

Maybe, like our own commercial society, an aspect of their trade-oriented civilization was to put on a happy face, the

121

playful art only insulating something sinister. The phantoms that lay between how the culture appeared and what actually went on have been quietly haunting. Maybe writing about it now, with attention to the undercurrents, would make it possible to perceive something more.

Welcoming distraction on the overnight ferry to Crete, my companion, Steve, and I found ourselves talking with two other American couples. Not long into the evening, we adopted another traveller, an Aussie. Elaine was touring the world by herself. She had that same imperious manner all travellers from the British Empire seemed to share—unshakable confidence that the world was theirs to enjoy.

Long before arriving at the port of Iraklion, Steve and I invited the others to travel in our van, the seven of us having discovered that we were all intending to visit Knossos, a Minoan palace. Still baffled by the degree of my willingness to go-along-with-the-crowd in my previous venture in Turkey, I observed our group process with a certain hesitancy.

What I knew about Minoan art ever since first seeing it in art school prepared me to expect loving it without reservation. I'd always sensed that it held some heartfelt meaning unlike so much other art which could be appreciated only intellectually. Now, finally, I was going to see the real thing!

As colorful and straightforward as Egyptian painting, Minoan art is less stiff, reflecting the undulating quality of the surrounding turquoise sea—an integral aspect of this merchant civilization. Although on a map the island of Crete might appear isolated, it's location in the Mediterranean put it in the middle of watery highways connecting it with several significant civilizations. It was a natural crossroad between the raw materials of Europe and buyers in the Middle East and Egypt.

We arrived at Iraklion early in the morning and decided to go to Knossos immediately. According to a brochure, archaeologists dated the site from 3000 to 1150 B.C. Were they suggesting the building itself existed for almost 2000 years? As I pondered this question, one of the group, also reading from the brochure, told us that a nearby museum held artifacts from Knossos as well as from a number of other sites dating from the same period. We agreed to go there later in the day.

As early as we arrived at Knossos, it was already teeming with tourists. We entered the ruins, a combination of broken foundations and grand staircases leading to restored rooms with colorful frescoes. The palace meandered over a long rolling hill, perhaps being, as some archaeologists suggest, the labyrinth of Homer's legend of the Minotaur. But unlike dark caverns said to be inhabited by the monster son of King Minos, walking through this enchanting architecture now was far from fearful.

Even in partial reconstruction, there was a feeling of gaiety and grace, porches, staircases, air shafts, and clerestories bathing the chambers in light and air. Unusual pillars, wider at the top than at the bottom subtly suggested a sense of more substance coming from above than from below. Though I'd never seen them before, these were the kind of pillars I had put in one of my own temple sculptures!

Only when we approached the very top of the palace hill, my body heavy in the heat and arid sunlight, and in spite of the presence of other tourists, did I feel a sense of separation and loss. Here, surrounded only by sky, we came upon a huge stone sculpture of bull's horns several times our own height, surely a place of consecration. This common symbol of male potency seemed to be the counterpart of the fertile mother goddess that the Cretans worshipped.

King Minos is said to have been one of the offspring of Zeus, king of the gods, who in the form of a bull carried Europa to Crete where she bore him children. Homer wrote that Theseus, son of the Athenian King Aegeus, travelled here to stop the horror of an annual sacrifice of Athenian youths to the Minotaur. King Minos' daughter, Ariadne, fell in love with Theseus and gave him a ball of twine so he could find his way out of the labyrinth after slaying the monster.

Looking at frescoes of dolphins cavorting in the waves, or at the procession of handsome youths bearing offerings through a corridor, I simply rejected the dark myth of sacrifice, until the repetition of one image finally reawakened the sense of disquiet I had atop the palace hill. First, we saw it on a fresco at Knossos, then variations of it were restated again and again on vessels and clay seals at the museum—youths, both male and female, grasping the horns of a bull and leaping over its back. The innate danger of such an exercise finally brought to a halt my ability to dismiss the legend. Was this venture a sport, a daring rite, or a sacrificial ritual? It's never become clear to me, though there was never any depiction of bloodshed for bull or athlete.

Quickly tiring of the number of tourists in Iraklion, we agreed on wanting to go somewhere quieter. A recently excavated Minoan palace on the far eastern end of this long narrow island was appealing for its remoteness, knowing it was not yet developed for tourist trade. Eagerly driving through mountainous territory, we flinched at the sight of newly cut roads, appearing like red raw wounds in the lush landscape.

We periodically stopped at tavernas. Some were secluded meeting places, others more like general stores sometimes displaying a few trays of vegetable stews kept hot cafeteria-style. Never seeing any women inside, we behaved cautiously, understanding that our small group was crossing some kind of cultural barrier. The men we saw were tall, mustached, with an upright and robust bearing, all wearing beautifully embroidered back packs made of brightly-colored striped hand-woven fabric. Infrequently, we saw women walking in a field or doing errands near a village, always in black and covered from head to toe. Their scurrying made them appear bent and old. On occasion, we got close enough to see that even the young ladies looked this way, in sharp contrast to their sturdy men.

Never had I seen color such as this in a landscape. In addition to the clear Mediterranean light, it was winter which meant that it rained every ten or twenty minutes. Clouds scuttled through a cerulean blue sky and from our perch in the van atop the mountains we watched their shadows flicker across the otherwise sunlit landscape turning pale green herbs to dark green, dark green trees to black, flowerpot orange earth to saturated red-orange, grayish olive drab trees to deep green and all back to their original colors when the clouds passed. Dormant grape vine leaves were yellow and oranges were ripe on trees everywhere.

Eventually, we came to a little village called Epano (Upper) Zakros where, unlike the previous villages, the whitewashed houses were detached from each other. Next to each was a private garden filled with vegetable greenery and orange trees hung with fruit. Standing on the sidewalk we could hear water tinkling below us. Our self-appointed guide, apparently the only man in the village who spoke English or who was willing to speak with tourists, explained that the sound of the water was the mountain stream diverted through a mill that ground the town flour. Except for us, the village appeared eerily devoid of people. Were they hiding or was it just the time of day?

Our guide took us for a hike above the village. I seemed to be the only one disturbed about going into the wilderness with this unknown person. We walked alongside a little stream. As we climbed, he pointed out dozens of herbs used for cooking, medicine, and tea. There were thousands of plants indigenous only to Crete, he explained. Through the crystal clear water, we could see every plant and stone on the creek bed. Yet another beauty was its sound as it trickled over rocks and boulders, falling toward the sea.

We asked if there were any cottages for rent down on the beach. It's a Greek summer resort, he told us, empty at this time of year, except for one inn keeper and one tourist couple staying with him. He was sure we'd be able to rent a cottage. Just go to the inn and ask. The cluster of houses along the beach was called Kato (Lower) Zakros, he explained. Then, having received directions from him on how to continue on the road we came in on, the seven of us piled back into the van and proceeded.

This part of the mountain was horseshoe-shaped, its two ends dipping into the sea, closing the valley to outsiders, unless they came through Epano Zakros, as we had. The valley itself was relatively flat, used by the village for farming.

As we descended into it, I began to have new anxiety, which before long grew into unmistakable fear. Trying to find something to pin it on only added to my distress. I felt too foolish to even mention it, so incompatible were my worries with the beauty around us. Was I going crazy? Meanwhile, my van mates, oblivious to my misery, were chattering like happy monkeys.

This must be the Garden of Eden! Look at the color! Fields full of vegetables! Look, bananas over there!

Despite the splendor, still, I couldn't shake my apprehension, even while guardedly joining in to point out spots where the usually orange earth was, instead, dusty rose or violet.

Not more than twenty minutes later, we arrived at the shore. The water was serene, azure. To the north, in the Mediterranean was a low cone-shaped island. To either side of us, at a distance, were the ends of the mountain descending into the water. White-painted cement block cottages were pleasantly spaced and had the undemanding aspect of vacation huts.

Mark, who spoke Greek, arranged for us to rent a cottage. The innkeeper introduced us to the tourists staying with him. Also from Chicago, just a little older, they nevertheless took what seemed to be an almost parental interest in all we were doing. As if I knew them from home, their presence provided a momentary sense of security.

We bought food on market day at a nearby village when farmers brought their produce from miles around. Our shared cooked meals were work-intensive—stews like the Greek food we ate in the tavernas, complex combinations of vegetables, flavored with local herbs, apples, and small amounts of meat used as a condiment. Still on guard, even while we were swimming and walking, I was able to relax only during the preparation of meals.

Waist high in the corner, a simple fireplace was designed specifically for cooking. Two ledges next to each other on the same level were ingeniously contrived with a few inches of space between them. Sticks were laid for fire in this opening and the cooking pot set over it. The chimney was a rounded organic form like adobe, a work of sculpture in itself. The sink didn't have running water. Instead, on the wall above it hung a small decorative metal tank with a tap near the bottom. We filled it with water pumped from a well out back and carried to the house in a bucket. In the counter, what looked like a sink had a drain that flowed out onto the sandy beach.

Now would be a good time to sew a dress, I decided, and bought some subtly printed brushed fabric at the market. In the evening, after we'd eaten, while my companions made music and chatted in the kerosene lamplight, I listened to them, sewing by hand without a pattern. It felt calming and of the essence.

In the midst of this beautiful simplicity and companionship, I continued keeping vigil, for my strange misgivings were never far away. My normal state was one of anxiety, yet it was impossible to pin on our surroundings why I was experiencing such a heightened version of it. I told no one my fears. If they were to make fun of me, my need to find a cause would only escalate.

Walks along the shore, taken to quiet myself, instead caused me to think that the land seemed not very far above the water, making the sea feel threatening in spite of it's gentle lapping. Maybe there were unknown strangers prowling around nearby, Greeks who resented young American tourists. I spotted goats leaping nimbly among the rocks and speculated, Might there be more dangerous animals? Was that what my sense of danger was coming from?

The palace we had come here to see turned out to be quite near the cottages, but there was simply not much to look at. The walls had totally crumbled and no restoration had been done. There were no beautiful murals, no rooms to enter or stairways to descend. All that was apparent was a foot or two of foundation and the indication of many small rooms. Compared to Knossos, there was little substance. We had heard rumors that what had been most remarkable were the objects found inside the rubble, many still intact and carted off to museums for study. Despite the utter destruction of the buildings, a clear picture of daily life 1500 B.C. had been revealed. I continued to hope that our disappointment and my apprehension would be offset by the beauty there.

A couple of days into our stay, Elaine wandered off to refresh herself by exploring the valley on her own. She was still gone long after we expected her to be back. The others began to question her absence, too. Was my fear a premonition about her? We agreed to start searching, all six of us hiking in the direction she mentioned intending to go. After about half an hour, we met her on her way back. She had walked all the way out to one end of the horseshoe.

It's much further away than it looks, she told us.

The next day, after commenting to the innkeeper about the large snails we saw everywhere, he told us they were edible. We collected some for dinner, putting them in a couple of paper sacks and leaving them in the kitchen. By the time we returned from our afternoon's exploration, the snails had dispersed themselves all over the cottage. It took almost as much effort to collect them again as when they had been outside. For the next couple of hours we continued finding them everywhere—on the ceiling, under the beds, inside a shoe, behind the furniture. We bravely cooked them, realizing in our greedy enthusiasm for free food that we had prepared and then ate way too many. Were we all going to fall ill?

Did you notice the canyon? Mark asked.

It sliced right through the horseshoe and could be entered directly from the valley floor. The others decided to take a walk through it. I, as usual, followed reluctantly. Fairly narrow, it was making me feel a bit claustrophobic. Here, the remarkable shapes of its walls were beautifully sculpted by the ferocity of water that had, at some time in the past, run through it.

Hints of caves were too high in the walls for us to be able to tell whether they were just deep indentations or actually led into the interior of the mountain. As we proceeded, I kept expecting to be confronted by a stranger or an animal or something that would prove our vulnerability. Even in this almost barren part of the terrain, scrubby plants, looking and smelling like herbs had taken a foothold in every crevice they could. A couple of hours later, when we completed our walk, I was relieved to return to the expansiveness of the valley.

After nine days of my exhausting amazement and foreboding, we bid good-bye to the tourists at the inn, driving back to the ferry that would return us to Athens. Nothing bad had happened. Would I ever understand why I felt so fearful in that beautiful place?

Before leaving Crete, at another market, I purchased a couple of clay sculptures, small enough to be held in hand. They were vessel-like forms, with scenes of animals and people inside. When I imagined showing them to friends back home, I knew they would think I had made them, the art looking so much like my own sculptures.

Seven months in Europe and the Middle-East, I finally arrived home, still seeking direction in my life. There were no obvious signs or situations like those that had led me to taking the trip. Now, mostly, I was digesting, feeling that a picture of my psyche must look like the Little Prince's boa that swallowed an elephant.

My friends and I were having a celebratory party for the

furniture-painting shop I recently opened where bright enamel colors cheered dreary old wooden items found cheap in junk stores. My oldest friend, Stef, said while handing me a shiny-jacketed new book, Here's something about Crete. It was a book review edition from the newspaper where she worked.

The cover photo was of a sculpted bull's head sporting golden horns. My eyes must have been bugging out of my face as I read the title, *Zakros: The Discovery of a Lost Palace of Ancient Crete*.[1] Did she realize she'd found a book about the exact place I'd been?

When everyone left, I finally had a chance to examine it. Excitedly, I riffled through the pages. My exhilaration grew as I turned the page to a map of the valley, recognizing the shape of the land. The author told about the history of the archaeological excavation itself. Over a period of at least a hundred years, sporadic finds by peasants farming the area occasionally aroused interest. The isolation of the east end of Crete, with few and difficult roads through the mountainous terrain helped keep the secret. Although the most recent dig had occurred in the 60s, just a few years before my trip, the site had been identified as archaeologically significant as early as 1852, with the first systematic excavation having begun in 1901.

That excavation, however, was interrupted by torrential rains sweeping away over 4,000 trees, flooding most of the cultivated land. Rushing waters had carried away such masses of earth and boulders as to threaten the lives of the excavators. Was it this violence that belied the beauty we had found there? The book went on to say that before the rains had begun, the remains of a dozen buildings had been revealed as well as other scattered structures. Considerable quantities of household and workshop items indicated there were many more riches to be found. Nevertheless, it was sixty years before the investigation was renewed!

I continued flipping pages frantically, unable to keep my attention on the documentation of building layouts or the cataloguing of items found in a series of workrooms. Reading a paragraph here, a picture description there, I learned that the palace and houses, upon excavation, revealed that their devastation was just as sudden and far more pervasive to human property than that which ended the 1901 dig. This area had been repeatedly inundated; though, by far the worst damage known was the destruction of the ancient palace and town.

Workshops, kitchens, supply halls containing all their storage jars, foods being prepared for meals, raw materials and tools being used in the workshops of artisans were buried, all found where they had been left. The lack of skeletons indicated there was enough warning for people to get out before the complete collapse of several levels of building above these rooms sealed them for thousands of years. Furthermore, the severity of the destruction and lack of plundering indicated that all this damage was solely from calamitous natural disaster, not invasion. Not even the people who had lived there had been able to plunder it. What had happened to them? Were they washed out to sea? The characteristic pottery provided clear evidence dating the event at 1450 B.C.

A photo of the ravine grabbed my eye. I read that when there were heavy rains, water washed through it in torrents connecting it with a river that, over the years had often changed its bed as it ran through the valley, requiring the farmers to reassign cultivating fields or remove huge piles of gravel and rock. This canyon, called by the archaeologists the Gorge of the Dead, contained a large quantity of ancient burial sites within its walls. We had been walking through a vertical graveyard that, to this day, periodically flooded suddenly and violently!

Although evidence indicated that other important centers in central and eastern Crete were simultaneously damaged by a series of catastrophic earthquakes and fires, the final annihilation at Zakros was the eruption of the volcano north of Crete. The island Thera sank by two-thirds. Some of the resulting tsunamis were documented as having carried ships from Cretan ports to as far as a kilometer inland. Protected Zakros harbor and the encircling character of the mountains might very well have contained and concentrated the violent tsunami water.

While the archaeology at Knossos indicated another half to three centuries of occupation, the devastation at Zakros and the other Cretan centers was complete, coinciding with the end of Minoan society. From this time, the already burgeoning pre-Greek Mycenaean culture descending from northern Greece became dominant and all that was further seen of Minoan artifacts came from remnants left in distant places where they had traded.

I grabbed *The Horizon Book of Lost Worlds*[2] from my bookshelf and opened it up to Crete, not sure what I was looking for in such a hurry. Scanning the pages, I discovered a story about Sir Arthur Evans, renowned for his archaeological explorations of Knossos. While there in 1926, he wrote in his journal about experiencing an earthquake which lasted a minute and a quarter. Already in bed, with some trepidation, he, nevertheless, decided to stay in his basement bedroom, trusting the strength of the construction of his house. The movement, which felt like a ship in a storm began to have the same physical effects on him in spite of the short duration of time. The single bell at his house began to ring and he could also hear distant church bells jangling. A muffled roar began to arise and he was reminded of how the ancients had described earthquakes as being caused by a bull tossing the earth on its horns. The sound emanating from deep within the earth, he wrote, astounded him by how much it was like the eerie bellowing of a bull.

1. Charles Scribner's Sons, New York, 1969.
2. American Heritage Publishing Co., Inc, New York, 1962.

-end-

Return to Lake Charles, Louisiana

As an adolescent I aspired to lasting fame,
I craved factual certainty,
and I thirsted for a meaningful vision of human life—
so I became a scientist.
This is like becoming an archbishop so you can meet girls.

- M. CARTMIL

"Hand me my Listerine—and don't give me that look," Berry said, "I'm afraid my breath smells from garlic in the soup Kathryn brought."

"It doesn't," I tried to reassure her as I walked around the bed to retrieve the bottle from her cabinet drawer. Against orders, I also brought a cup for her to spit into. Sometimes she would use it and sometimes, as on that day, she'd just swallow the disinfectant while holding me in a rebellious gaze.

Having gotten what might have been her declaration of independence out of the way, we dove into discussion, first rehashing the story of Crete. Berry had laughed at my description of our discovering snails hidden everywhere and I was glad to have finally written at least one episode with a little humor in it.

There had actually been one more foreboding incident, but, Berry insisted it be removed. "Too much," she concluded. I depended on her judgment as to whether it was overkill. All I could see was that it was true. Perhaps it put too much emphasis on other people. Mark's girlfriend Paula had stepped on a nail and within hours an angry red streak showed under the skin from her heel to halfway up her calf. She was visibly shaken and we were scared for her, too. Again, I wondered if this event would prove to be the cause of my psychological distress. However, Mark took her to Epano Zakros where a female doctor cleaned the wound and gave Paula a tetanus shot. By the next day, the streak was gone. Although Berry had me cut that story, she did allow the last menacing tale about the walk through the canyon.

Berry then said, seemingly out of nowhere, "I don't like quo-

133

tation marks. They're too fussy. I always structured dialogue without using them."

I hadn't had much conversation in any of the stories so I just followed her lead. Maybe that's why she hadn't mentioned them much except in establishing not using them in her memoirs. Most of my writing dealt with sorting out an interior world that was only sporadically confirmed by the outer one. When deliberating about my bewilderment on Crete, Berry said again, "You're psychic."

"The events never seem as clear to me as the way people who call themselves 'psychic' describe their experiences. They give dates, name names, describe circumstances, are so confident. I think we all have as much 'sensitivity' as I have. Like in the Cretan story, there I was working so hard to describe nothing more than a pressing feeling that eventually got explained through no understanding of my own. The answer was just handed to me, literally, handed to me in a book." Berry looked thoughtful but said nothing.

We were still working on her memoirs, she frequently telling me the thoughts she had been having about them at night.

"I often write during the night," she said, "since I don't sleep much. Write and pray. There's really nothing more to do. Last night I was contemplating a job that Darrell once had with a wholesale grocer. It didn't last very long, though. He had noticed a motto on the letterhead, 'Better Than The Best And As Good As The Rest. Laughing robustly, he called on the owner, announcing that it needed to be changed. His continuing laughter, I suppose, didn't help persuade."

"What happened?"

"I'm afraid he was sent home early that day with a partial paycheck and an equally reduced reputation.

"There was more," Berry said. "He'd been employed during Thanksgiving by this company and had been given a live turkey. Imagine coming into the kitchen to prepare breakfast and finding, chained to the leg of the stove, this creature staring you down. Darrell always had to do the dirty work, so I imagine he's the one who killed and de-feathered it."

"I feel sorry for him," I said, shaking my head, "required at such a young age to be the man of the house."

"He was incorrigible. You can understand his becoming a lawyer. At his next job, he paid no attention to the dictation—examined the facts himself, wrote the reply, and expected his boss to sign the letter. Even as a young child he would correct me in my reading to him from the comics. From my viewpoint I was improving the story. From his, I was simply erroneous."

Berry explained that with both of the youngsters making better incomes, the family was able to move into larger quarters and eventually regain possession of some of their old belongings from home.

"To complete our image, Mama sent me to distress sales where I could buy bric-a-brac and other accouterments of the rich." Then she paused, "Can we stop here? I'm feeling too tired to go on."

"Sure, I'm sorry, I didn't realize..."

"You can't always know." She pressed her hand to her head and then relaxed. She once explained it was a shooting pain but never mentioned it again. She rarely discussed any of her symptoms. "Take some more money for sauerkraut," she added, handing me the basket. When I lifted the plastic container it rattled. I peered into it, then raised my head to meet her eyes. She grinned. "I've been saving my pain pills—just in case."

"Don't...don't you need them all?" I stammered. I could sympathize with Berry's unspoken plan, having often thought about what I would do if I were in her situation. Nevertheless, it frightened me to have her allude to it.

I had read *Last Wish* by Betty Rollin, a controversial true story about Rollin's elderly mother in the terminal stages of a slow painful cancer. She had asked her daughter to help her die. A few years later, I'd read *One True Thing*, a novel by Anna Quindlen based on the same concept with the additional element of a trial for mercy killing and two family members who each think the other did it. With my known antipathy for the medical system, my recent run-in at After-Care, and my not knowing Berry until recently, I thought I'd make a perfect scapegoat if there were anything questionable about her death.

The Black Monk*

Why is it not necessary to doubt?
Because it is not necessary to have certainty.
- J.G. BENNETT

When I told Berry that I didn't much like short stories, she said, "You just haven't found the right ones for you. I think you'll feel differently about Chekhov. Have you read his story, *The Black Monk?*"

The little library in Charles Town had the tale in a collection. A man named Kovrin hallucinates a legendary monk dressed in black, entering into hopeful enlightening conversations with him. Kovrin is happy, filled with energy, feeling special and with a sense of purpose. However, at one point, the monk says,

> "I am a phantom."
> "Then you don't exist?" said Kovrin.
> "You can think as you like," said the monk, with a faint smile. "I exist in your imagination, and your imagination is part of nature, so I exist in nature."
> "You have a very old, wise, and extremely expressive face, as though you really had lived more than a thousand years," said Kovrin. "I did not know that my imagination was capable of creating such phenomena. But why do you look at me with such enthusiasm? Do you like me?"
> "Yes, you are one of those few who are justly called the chosen of God. You do the service of eternal truth. Your thoughts, your designs, the marvelous studies you are engaged in, and all your life, bear the Divine, the heavenly stamp, seeing that they are consecrated to the rational and the beautiful—that is, to what is eternal."
> "You said 'eternal truth.' ...but is eternal truth of use to man and within his reach, if there is no eternal life?"
> "There is eternal life," said the monk.
> "Do you believe in the immortality of man?"
> "Yes, of course. A grand, brilliant future is in store for you men. And the more there are like you on earth, the sooner will this future be realized. Without you who serve the higher principle and live in full understanding and freedom, mankind would be of little account;

developing in a natural way, it would have to wait a long time for the end of its earthly history. You will lead it some thousands of years earlier into the kingdom of eternal truth—and therein lies your supreme service. You are the incarnation of the blessing of God, which rests upon men."

"And what is the object of eternal life?" asked Kovrin.

"As of all life—enjoyment. True enjoyment lies in knowledge, and eternal life provides innumerable and inexhaustible sources of knowledge, and in that sense it has been said: 'In my Father's house there are many mansions.'"

"If only you knew how pleasant it is to hear you!" said Kovrin, rubbing his hands with satisfaction.

"I am very glad."

* http://chekhov2.tripod.com/index.htm
201 Stories by Anton Chekhov, translated by Constance Garnett

Kovrin's family, concerned about his disordered mind, sends him to get help. When "cured" he becomes cruel, irritable and uninteresting. He destroys the lives of those closest to him, ignores his own developing tuberculosis, yet dies with a smile on his face because in the throes of death he sees the monk in black once again.

I told Berry about looking at some synopses after reading it. "They seem to focus on material interpretations—Kovrin's insanity, how delusive and destructive his thinking. One summary also referred to Chekhov's own death from TB after years of obsessive work and travel as if he were only writing about himself."

"Maybe he was,' she said in a tone that didn't limit the possibilities, and then she added, "Would the story have the staying power it has if it didn't speak to a paradox that we, in this culture, sense but don't address about the nature of reality?"

Watershed Experiences

All societies need their gifted ones, their artists and mystics:
without them, the land becomes weary and disenchanted....
When the music of enchantment ceases to sound, chaos returns.
  - CAITLIN AND JOHN MATTHEWS, ENCYCLOPEDIA OF CELTIC WISDOM

Still conforming to routine, alternating visiting Berry with filling in
for Collette at the library two days a week, I usually arrived at the
nursing home early in the morning with hummus, which she had
reinstated as her food of choice. I detached the stubborn foil seal
from the top, watched her dig in as I pulled the curtain around her
bed, moved the breakfast tray over to the sink, muted the TV, and
plugged in my laptop, all while we greeted each other with the latest news.

In Berry's memoirs, she was still describing her employment.
At work she had plenty of time to daydream and flirt with the
handsome men who frequented the bank.

"I left my fairy godfathers alone thinking them to be in a special category. However, that soon ended when Mr. Knapp had me
sitting on his lap regularly in the dark of the board of directors'
room. It was innocent enough and the locked door prevented anyone from walking in on us. Continuing this activity after hours,
however, I would not allow as I was given seven-and-a-half minutes to arrive home after the bank's closing time.

"I remember only one instance where my daydreaming caused
trouble. So oblivious to it at the time, I am hard pressed now to
imagine how I bypassed humiliation."

"What happened?"

"By this time I was a fully qualified stenographer. Late one
afternoon, there was a flurry to meet a deadline on a ten-page legal
document for the Reconstruction Finance Corporation. All the
trustees had signed it and I was asked to put my John Henry on it
as witness. Lost in my musings, I did precisely what I was told. In
sudden silence, everyone standing there quickly reconvened in the
board room without me. Someone was sent to retype the last page.

That done, the trustees were gathered, once again, to sign."

When Berry dictated the story, I pointed out how she never said directly what she had done.

"I think it's good to be elliptical," she explained.

"Elliptical?"

"Yes, you have to give the reader credit for being able to fill in some of the gaps themselves. It's more fun for them, more engaging. Don't you like figuring some things out for yourself when you're reading?" she asked.

"I don't remember noticing. When I was writing the newsletter, we felt compelled to explain everything."

"Yes, those well-designed declarative sentences have been your biggest stumbling block."

I smiled. Berry always balanced her criticism of my writing with a kind word. It did make it easier to hear. But knowing how sharp she could be, those tendernesses still awoke in me a sense of danger. Not as often as they used to, though.

When we had been winding up my story about Crete, Berry asked how it was I had decided to go to Europe.

"Oh, there were a whole series of coincidences that led to my going...hmmm...maybe that should be the next story we work on—my friendship with Roy, beginning in high school. He was the main incentive for going even though he had died five years before."

Berry was attentive.

"He had been so many things to me," I said, catapulted into talking about him.

While I described our meeting in the high school orchestra, Berry was trying to move the sausage-shaped pillow without breaking my stream of thought. I stood up, still chatting, and helped her push it down further under her back.

Then she pressed the side of her head in that characteristic gesture she made toward a passing wave of pain. With effort, she rolled on her side, propping herself up onto her right elbow.

Watching her search for a comfortable position, I finally interrupted myself, asking, "Is there something I can do?"

"Would you lower the bed a little?"

As I cranked it down, I resumed talking about Roy.

"Do you have a photograph?"

I had to think. Did I?... "The yearbook! I'll bring it next time." Trying to picture him at that age, I wondered, after all this time, whether my memory would match the photo.

Unexpectedly, telling Berry about Roy was stirring up old grief—for the despairing girl of my youth, for Roy's short life, and, perhaps new grief, for Berry who, as she did that day, was more often saying things like, "I'd leave if I could be sure my work here were finished." Then, referring specifically to me, she added, "I think you can write on your own now. You know what's important."

"How would you be sure about your work being finished?" I asked, hoping to make her less sure.

"Well, that's the trouble. I still find life so interesting," she said almost lamenting. Returning to Roy, she asked me to tell her more. Writing the story over a period of several weeks, I started with what I'd told Berry that day. We talked more than usual during these readings. She seemed to be as impressed by him as I had been.

"He was so wise for his age," she would say repeatedly. As we discussed the many subjects Roy introduced me to, I was reminded of the scope of experiences he gave me. Often, they were ordinary things—like pointing out how to see distant rain falling from the clouds or introducing me to pomegranates. How many years would have passed before I'd have eaten one? These thoughts reawakened my gratitude toward him. I hadn't told Berry all of Roy's story, though, saving the end for the written version.

The Fourth Story—Roy

...there are those phases when hot leads
and fresh evidence pop up all over the place,
convincing you beyond a doubt that
magic is one of the fundamental properties of reality.

- ROB BREZSNY

Roy

In the six years I had known Roy, he had been my buddy, mentor, lover, and good friend, again. Eventually, I think he became a guiding spirit although I didn't quite believe it but had to say it anyway.

I'd met him in orchestra. In high school, orchestra was a godsend. Throughout my childhood I had always found any kind of change difficult, including the transition from a neighborhood elementary school to a high school with 3,600 students. Everything conspired to make the change in my life gloomy. The older neighborhood where Senn High was located was shabby by comparison, full of huge dreary apartment buildings, dirty streets, and distraught-looking people.

Instead of walking a block to get there, we had to ride two buses on public transportation. Mid-year graduation meant beginning the new experience by waiting at the bus stop on icy streets in the middle of winter. We'd be bundled from our toes to our eyeballs—boots, coats, hats, mittens, and mufflers to fight the bone-chilling Chicago wind. I used to carry an umbrella just to block the gusts on my way home. Without the device, turning the corner into the north wind would literally knock the breath out of me.

At school, while my friends were assigned to home rooms and classes with each other, I was placed in a home room that had no one from my grammar school. Not a single one of my friends were in any of my classes. To make matters worse, home room was filled with poor achievers who were often in

141

trouble. I despaired when I found out that assignment to it was for all four years of school and had been determined by our recent IQ tests. I had been placed with my supposed equals. It was devastating to my already-faltering identity. Misery provided the impetus to go weeping to a school counselor. She adjusted my schedule to have lunch and at least a couple of the nine class periods with people I knew.

When an older cousin recommended taking orchestra instead of music appreciation, most of my little clique joined me. The idea of making music rather than thinking about it must have appealed to all of us. That impulsive decision changed my life.

Because orchestra was considered geeky, it was the one place where all the idiosyncratic kids could gather. We had a good time, laughing a lot with no intent of hurting anyone. A year of orchestra class and private cello lessons prepared us to join the school symphony. There were a hundred members, many of them planning to study music in college. Those kids were really good, carrying the rest of us.

There was no aspect of my life Roy didn't touch. To this day I'm often reminded that I first heard about some particular topic from him. Yet, he never lectured or pressed me to be different from who I was. He was just interested in everything and enthusiastic about sharing what he learned.

He played the clarinet over in the wind section. It wasn't his looks as much as it was his sense of humor and the expression on his face that drew me—his eyes wide open to the world, his easy nature enthusiastically taking it in. Not that he wasn't kind of handsome, too—black hair and owlish glasses. As far away as he sat from us cellos, it took a good part of the year to attract his friendship.

His remarkable mind and adventurous spirit also provided me with badly needed guidance which I wasn't getting from home. What he had to say about responding to life's endless challenges always made sense. Two years ahead in school, Roy kept in contact when he graduated only a year after we met.

He attended the University of Illinois downstate.

There was something about Roy that made the fluctuations of my external world less threatening. I was like a bird ready to flee in response to the slightest movement. Yet, I kept up an appearance of composure that held my burgeoning frenzy in check.

It didn't make sense. Although change promised a way out of inner chaos, still, the thought of it felt fraught with danger. It seemed a necessity, however, if one hoped for a transformed world.

Since the Art Institute didn't have mid-year entrance when I graduated, Roy encouraged me to go to Roosevelt University in the spring and get a head start on electives. He said that Roosevelt attracted an unusual student body—Korean War veterans and experienced older people. I did as he advised, finding the students forward thinking and interesting, just as he said. In comparison, when I later met the art students, they were competitive and seemingly disinterested in anything besides their careers.

In the autumn, having returned to Chicago, Roy suggested that I move into the skyscraper dorm where he was living. This gave us the opportunity to spend more time together. I think he hoped, by directing my attention away from home, to deflect my futile attempts to win parental approval.

He took me camping for the first time in my life, cooking a juicy steak over the campfire. Could anything taste so good? After eating, we lay back and watched the moon through the trees. Look how the full moon is bright enough to cast shadows, he said. I'd never seen that before.

With both of us living at the dorm, we saw each other at least a couple of times a week, meanwhile each of us dating other people. We just hung out together—going for a walk or seeing a movie.

Every meeting with Roy seemed to lead to a new experience, usually pleasant—the bagel bakery at two in the morning or the take-out joint he discovered hidden away among five-story factories and warehouses. It was open late at night in an area with no other retail shops. How had he found it? They sold freshly cooked french-fried shrimp served up in a paper bag, a whole pound with the most delicious sauce for a price even students could afford. No indoor seating. If we wanted to eat them hot, we'd have to eat right there in the car on the street, watching the moon rise over the lake.

Roy introduced me to the works of e.e. cummings, Ferlinghetti, T.S. Eliot, and Japanese haiku poetry, his obvious enjoyment making them come alive. While having no difficulty accepting the abstractions of modern art, I was thoroughly intimidated by the possibility of misinterpreting words. Mystified, Roy asked, Where'd that come from? English is so direct.

At home, where no one seemed to understand what I was talking about, I thought the problem must come from not using the right words. He helped me realize it was my feelings that were misunderstood.

Haiku poetry—a concrete spiritual sense conveyed by strong visual descriptions of the material world—interested me most.

The Great Buddha! Not at all does he blink an eyelid—as the hailstones fall.*

or:

Up the barley rows, stitching, stitching them together, a butterfly goes.*

* An Introduction to Haiku, Harold G. Henderson, Doubleday Anchor Books, 1958.

Roy's telling me about Steinbeck's *Cannery Row* and D.H. Lawrence's *Lady Chatterly's Lover* started me reading novels that described the paradoxes of human nature and society.

On my first visit to Roy's parents, I was astonished by his

mother. She was unpleasant to be around, talking at him aimlessly, questioning him without ever listening to his answers. Equally shocking as her behavior, though, was seeing how much he looked like her in spite of her plumpness and dutch-boy haircut. Fine black hair, pale translucent skin, high forehead, moon-round eyes—it was eerie, making me wonder fearfully, if he would one day begin to act like her.

As intrusive as she was, his father was almost ghostlike, downcast and restrained. He's a Buddhist, Roy explained, strange for a Jewish man of that generation. However, the topic of Buddhism opened the door for Roy to introduce me to concepts such as acceptance and detachment, the practice of meditation, and the writer Herman Hesse. We also talked about Taoism, putting into words ideas that my mind had already begun grappling with about living in harmony with the natural order.

The skyscraper dorm we lived in belonged to Northwestern University's medical and nursing schools. They rented out unoccupied rooms to students from other colleges. When pranks got out of hand—tossing water balloons out of seventh story windows—the students tried to pin blame on Roy and me. It never stuck but their mean-spiritedness inspired my moving out in the middle of winter to share an apartment with a girl from the Art Institute.

Determined to live within my means, I ate little but bread, which turned out to be a quick path to the chronic tonsillitis that had plagued me every winter of my life. More painful than I'd ever experienced, this time I could see a peculiar gray membrane covering my throat. The diagnosis was strep and mononucleosis. Exhausted by the sheer effort needed to keep functioning, I fell into hospital like it was a resort. Even the food tasted good.

Over my protests, the doctor insisted drugs were needed to make it less painful to eat. My tearful complaints the next day about a steady stream of visitors, mail deliveries throughout the night, and a giant staircase in the desert with a fried egg slinking down it finally persuaded him I might be able to eat without the assistance of codeine.

Roy brought me a book by Adele Davis. I learned from it that the bouts of acute shakiness and sudden tears I'd experienced since childhood might be caused by incorrect nutrition. This is how he launched my interest in learning about alternative methods of healing. I was so weak that I was unable to return to school full time. Then I was glad to have taken some of those academic requirements at Roosevelt.

After Roy's graduation from college, he went to veterinary school in Seattle, our correspondence a steady stream of silly, affectionate letters. He always visited when home. We'd have long discussions on the meaning of life, the influence of culture, the nature of thinking, topics that scared away most other people. During vacations he would invariably find something new to experience—working as a night clerk at a resort, driving a Good Humor ice cream truck, fishing in Alaska— always meeting people whose backgrounds were different from his.

On one of his visits home, something changed. There was an energy between us that made me want to touch him. We were resting on the stairs of my porch. Sitting one step below him, I laid my head on his thigh. He played with my hair silently.

Finally, he spoke, I don't know if I should say this or not. I like you more than as a platonic friend.

By this time we were standing. I put my arms around his waist and we embraced.

I couldn't look at you tonight, he continued, because I wanted to grab you but you can't go around grabbing your platonic friends. After all, if you can't trust a platonic friend, who are you going to trust?

Not delving into that question any further, we remarked on the strange turn of events but mostly hugged and kissed, enjoying being near each other for the short time he was home from Seattle.

Two weeks before he was to finish his final semester at veterinary school, I received a panic-stricken phone call from him. He was in Hawaii! Why had he run off so close to graduation? He didn't know. But after a few days of serious self-questioning he phoned again, confessing that he really wanted to be a medical doctor. He thought he could avoid becoming the arrogant and money-grubbing stereotype of a Jewish doctor by becoming a vet instead. Finally coming to terms with this, he applied to a pre-med program at the University of Illinois Chicago Campus and was accepted to begin the following fall. He'd be coming back to town!

Just before the semester began, Roy told me how excited and scared he was. I'd never heard him admit to being fearful of anything. Being a fantastic dreamer, he said, he had always been afraid that if he were to add any amount of certainty to his life he would lose his power to dream. How prescient!

By this time I was in love with David, a student from the Art Institute, sure that he was the man I would marry. In medical school, Roy, too, fell in love. Mary was a student in his pre-med class. Her strict father controlled all of her social activities. Taking pity on them, I would go with Roy to pick her up, pretending to be part of a group outing. Then they would drop me off and spend the evening alone together. She was even more vulnerable than I, I thought. Later on, she being unable or unwilling to commit to Roy, he began dating others. Nevertheless, as in his relationship with me, they remained close friends.

Then tragedy struck. Larry, Roy's roommate phoned me.

Roy has a broken leg, he said, sounding peculiarly panicky.

How did he do it? I asked.

He was just walking through the apartment, Larry explained. That's when I laughed, unable to grasp what had happened.

Roy later said that he couldn't remember a time, even as a child, when he didn't have pain in that leg. It turned out that cancer had eaten away at the bone and the cancerous break was too close to his hip for amputation.

When I visited, Mary often was there, too. After one of his biopsies, Roy was being given an IV which he wanted removed. Trying to convince hospital staff to remove it, he kept telling them he wasn't hungry anymore.

When, after eating a meal, they still hadn't removed it, Mary said, They undoubtedly have some drug in there.

Roy asked, Why would they be giving me a drug?

I don't know, answered Mary, maybe there's something wrong with you. And we all laughed.

The doctors treated the cancer aggressively, trying several experimental drugs, but it wasn't long before cancer was found in his lungs. I hoped we'd be able to talk about death. I needed to talk about it, but he was afraid of upsetting me, Mary explained. Why was *she* telling me that?

I didn't know how to ask Roy to talk with me. In the past, he always just did. I was jealous of Mary for that, but I had my own great love, David, didn't I?

One visit, Roy was telling us how sorry he was for having asked Karen, his latest girlfriend up in Wisconsin, to marry him, thinking now that he shouldn't have been so weak as to bring her into this situation.

When I get out of here, let's all live together. You and Mary are the only two women I could live with. You could do whatever you want. We'd just live together!

Periodically, the three of us would hold hands and Mary and I would exchange caresses with Roy. Mary coolly took breaks to file her nails and comb her hair, getting ready for a date. We all joked and laughed at our own wisecracks about death.

Roy said, When I get out of here I'll take you both out to dinner, then added, Actually, you're the only ones I could marry, but I'd have to marry both of you.

Mary said, Roy, we can't fall in love, we know too much about each other. I thought again about my boyfriend. I loved him. And I loved Roy. I *wanted* to live with Roy. Was it promiscuous to think like that? Karen was his girlfriend now, and Mary was dating others. But, his words were a sincere expression of his love for us and I loved him. These thoughts were baffling only when I tried to figure how this could all work out.

Although I wanted to be with him more before he died, my fears of traveling across the city to his parents's house or of arousing jealousy in my boyfriend stopped me. Roy had requested only once that I come there. I soon regretted not having visited more, for, within two months, he was dead at the age of twenty-three.

At the funeral chapel service, when I began to cry speaking with his father, he shushed me. I thought his Buddhism was not detachment, but an excuse for denial. He was not going to let his emotions out or anyone else's in. Wouldn't that cause him more pain in the long run? Wasn't it unfair to Roy, to himself, to all of us who loved Roy?

Still rejoicing in my flourishing new love at school and, at least, in having known Roy, I wasn't at first that sensitive to the loss. I was used to intervals of separation. It hit more deeply as time went on, when I would feel desolate without the rhythm of our expected periods of togetherness. It was hard to believe I'd known him for only six years, yet I'd come to take his presence in my life for granted, like family or something more.

Almost a year before his leg broke, we had spoken about having been so many things to each other. He said, If we're not married by thirty we may as well marry each other. After all, if we persist in going through all the ups and downs of our lives, there'd be no reason we couldn't just continue.

After Roy's death, what did I do? I stayed in college to graduate with a masters degree while the man I thought to be the love of my life drifted away. Later, I taught part-time, worked as a graphic designer, and continued foundering through periods of confusion and doubt with no one to act as mentor. It's taken a lifetime for me to realize the importance of Roy's effect on me. Years of thinking to myself, I first heard about that from Roy, has driven home the magnitude of ideas and attitudes he educated me to.

As preoccupied as I was with every day living, the loss of Roy sounded a quiet drone in the background until my life took a particularly chaotic turn five years after his death. My companionable roommate decided to strike out on her own just at the time the three-story marble-halled, wainscoted apartment building we lived in across from Lincoln Park and close to the lake was sold to be razed and replaced by a lifeless skyscraper. Then I learned that the conglomerate that owned the company I worked for was using it as a tax write-off, purposely losing money. The owners had no intention of having us employees complete the business school franchise we were designing. Home and job were being pulled out from under me. I had to make some changes—soon.

It must have happened three or four days in a row. In the evening before bed I would think of a brilliant new plan to alter my existence and every morning I would awaken thinking about it, feeling sick to my stomach.

Then one morning I dreamed of Roy. He had a cast on his leg and was dressed in a white hospital gown, sitting up amidst white linens on a wide bed.

How do you *really* feel? I asked him. Silently, he held up an 8 1/2" x 11" paper, blank except for a finely-drawn equilateral cross in the very middle.

My face was pressed against the mattress and a voice was saying, This isn't a dream.

I repeated the words sleepily. This isn't a dream. This isn't a dream. Suddenly, wide awake, I sat up in bed. This isn't a dream!?

Immediately, I remembered my latest idea of what to do with my life—travel in Europe and see what I see. Don't set a return date. Maybe stay there. Fly Icelandic or take a Yugoslavian freighter—more of Roy's ideas from years back.

For the first time since I'd been trying to figure out what to do, I didn't feel sick to my stomach. Instead, I was excited, happy, feeling as if Roy were giving me encouragement. Usually over-anxious about anything new, having no clear idea how I'd go or who I'd go with didn't seem to be problems, just exciting blanks that needed to be filled in. The decision had already been made.

Still buzzing from the effects of my dream, that afternoon I went to an astrology lesson at a friend's apartment. It was the third class she was giving us, her workmates; and she was explaining the meaning of the astrological houses and planets.

Today, she said, I want to tell you something about the symbols used to designate the planets. To create the symbols, basic elements are combined in different ways which indicate the qualities of that planet. She began drawing at the top of a sheet of paper.

First, she explained, there's the circle, a symbol of spirituality. Then, drawing a crescent below, she said it was a symbol of potential. Lastly, there is the cross made up of two lines, the horizontal indicating the material world, the earth, and the vertical which traverses it, connecting heaven and earth. The cross, therefore, is a sign of bringing into our lives the latent spiritual forces we have within us.

Then, she slowly turned toward me smiling and held up the white paper for me to see with the circle and crescent at the top and the finely drawn equilateral cross right in the middle. With my mouth agape, I stared at her. I launched into a frenzied description of my daily attempts to solve the work and home dilemma, that morning's 'dream' about Roy surrounded by white, my asking what he *really* thought, his holding up the paper, the cross in the middle!

She laughed, "The universe seems to be making sure you get the message."

-end-

151

A Visit From Roy Once Again

Death is not extinguishing the light;
it is putting out the lamp because dawn has come.
- Rabindranath Tagore

One of the times Berry and I talked about Roy, I said, "I've been embarrassed and mystified by my laughter when Larry phoned to tell me about Roy's leg breaking. I don't know what that was about, just the absurdity of it breaking from no apparent cause. It reminds me of an incident in childhood when my closest friend's scary father bawled her out in front of me and she began to cry. I laughed. It seemed like a release of my fear of him as well as actually laughing at her. She had always been so bossy and never appeared vulnerable. Even at that age I was mortified by my multiple reaction."

"It's understandable," Berry said softly. "We're only supposed to feel one emotion at a time and it better be politically correct. I'm afraid we're more complex than we care to know."

During the time of writing about Roy, amidst my papers, I found an old letter of his and brought it to show Berry. Gloomily, I read about another feeling he and I shared.

> ...there exists a paradox about the true outsider, the one who always lives on the periphery of human activity, always has a part of him longing for the inside, to take part, but as soon as you get inside, everything is so stifling and restricted and responsibilities are heaped on you, that you can't stand it and out you go. Loneliness and freedom or companionship and restriction?

"I see he also had a gift for writing."

I nodded. "He had always given me so much, I've often wondered what he could possibly have received from me? Now I understand: I was so awed by him that I could let him be himself— no criticism, no demands. I never felt as if I had to hold onto him the way I did with other men.

"Before I ever met him, I had been on a quest to know the meaning of life. If I could understand why we were here, maybe I wouldn't feel so sad. My inner suffering and the outrages of human behavior that comprised the news were incomprehensible to me. Why should we live only to experience pain or purposeless violence? How could every religion claim to have the one true way and then persecute people who thought the same about their own religion? Roy kept me looking beyond the horizon."

"Yes, he seemed to have the long view of a much older man. He was unique, remarkably wise for his age." After a long silence, Berry surprised me, saying, "Such an important mentor, a genius. You should write a whole book about him to honor him."

Hearing her praise him pleased me, though the idea of writing a *book* on any topic seemed quite beyond something I could commit to.

Then, as if the thoughts were connected, Berry added, "Stop working for two weeks and don't come to see me during that time."

This aroused misgivings. The story was basically finished, but I refused to honor her second suggestion, thinking she might be planning to sneak off and die. Now, I believe she was hoping to die and trying to be kind to me.

I never did tell Berry that when I was in Europe, Roy came to mind a couple of times so strongly that it seemed as if I were being approached by him. The second time it happened, I got the notion he'd come to say good-bye, that he had some things to do and wouldn't be contacting me again for a long time, maybe never again during this lifetime. This wasn't my usual way of thinking.

Shortly after having finished Roy's story, I awoke in the middle of the night, recalling the emotion-packed dream that had awakened me.

I and a number of other people including Roy are visiting Berry. I haven't actually introduced them but he's talking with her already anyway. As I sit there, it slowly dawns on me—Roy isn't dead. How could I have thought he was dead? How could I have forgotten that he didn't die? Haven't I based my life on the belief that he died? I sit next to him, weeping. Knowing it's always been all right to cry around him, I continue, but, also, I don't want to. I'm confused and embarrassed that I could think he was dead when he was not. Why haven't I spent more time with him? And, finally, as if to distract me from this momentous revelation, I ask myself a question that propels me into wide-awake laughter, What will happen to my story?

When I described the dream to Berry, she smiled, nodding, saying only, "Yes...he's not dead."

I tried to let her words sink in.

Suddenly, I stopped smiling back at her. "Oh, Berry, I remember having the thought when Roy was first diagnosed, 'This will make a good story—Close Friend Dies Young.'"

"That's how it is to be creative. Most people think this kind of thinking is insensitive. It's just serpentine. You and I always have a lot of different thoughts at once. We notice them and admit it, even when some of them are not socially acceptable."

The dream was holding my confusion about death in front of me. In the afternoon, as I sat on the edge of my bed in our pleasantly sunlit bedroom at home, my mind drifted.

Oryx has me ride her across the veldt and then we stand around with the herd. I am apprehensive, looking around me restlessly. "Everything is fine," she says. "We aren't being stalked. Of greater concern, is your lack of belief that when death happens it is okay. Although you claim to want change, you always appear to do all you can to prevent it. As much as you believe in the continuing existence of the soul, you also are fearful it will not continue. You often claim to dislike something when its happening, but then you are fearful of leaving it for the unknown.

"At the same time, you are quick to give up to life-threatening situations which shows a deeply underlying belief in the eternal, don't you think? It's as if you're saying, 'Why struggle? Just get on

with the next step.' You're reluctant to put your actions behind your belief in the eternal, reluctant to give over your 'control' to the eternal who is quite willing to help."

I didn't know what to make of it. This didn't clarify anything except to expose all my inner contradictions.

Berry's Husband

The way to come to true sanity is just to see things as they are.
- J.G. BENNETT

Leaving aside talk about my old boyfriend, Berry told me about meeting her future husband, Randolf, who was renting a room across the street from her family's new digs. Her mother noticed that Randolf was smitten with Berry and suggested he take a room at their house. It wasn't long before he proposed marriage, which was accepted on the condition that Berry's mother approve of his family.

"His mother was a concert pianist. It never occurred to either Mama or me," Berry said smiling, "that his mother might disapprove of her only son marrying into what we believed to be near royalty."

Berry described a small rough patch before the impending marriage caused by Randolf's mother losing a necklace at their house and believing it stolen. However, it was discovered having fallen into a wastebasket next to the guest bedroom chest of drawers. Randolf and Berry were married before the war and when the Japanese attacked Pearl Harbor, Berry followed him, now in the army, to Texas. She said the prices of Christmas trees were so high that even with his officer status, they couldn't afford one.

"Randolf was so embarrassed about our not being able to afford a tree we'd been inspecting that he was about to purchase it anyway. I insisted we kidnap a nearby weed that was tall enough to substitute and string lights on it." Then she added, with her sly grin, "I don't think he was ever conscious of his disappointment in me during our thirty erotic years of marriage."

I smiled, easily believing there had once been a sensual and seductive Berry, in high contrast to her mayhem producing side.

After the war, they moved to New Orleans along with her mother and Darrell, now appearing to live in luxury because they could afford a grand apartment. "It cost $90 a month, which was a huge amount at the time."

"It must have been," I said, "I was paying that almost twenty years later!"

Berry said it was there, through nearly running over a woman who had been walking in the rain, that she met Dr. Fasting, the pedestrian's physician. Berry gloried in her good fortune. The doctor specialized in difficult medical cases. He diagnosed her mother and provided weekly treatments, essentially becoming the head of their family, worshipped by all.

"He really provided me a comprehensive liberal education and scholarly study of the Christian bible," Berry said. "I'm still grateful for his attentions."

She revealed, he eventually wanted to provide her with something even more. Yet, enamored as Berry was with him, she couldn't agree to the suggestion.

"What was your father like?" Berry asked one day.

How to describe him? His troubled face floated into my mind. "I feel sorry for him."

"Why?"

"He suffered so much. He worried about everything and never enjoyed anything besides comedies on television. Nor would he consider the possibility of learning how to stop worrying or to look for help. He was very unhappy and constantly let us know."

I told Berry that he was the affectionate one when I was little.

But he never talked with us, so, as my brother and I became more verbal, his ability to respond just kind of dried up. If we had been hurt at first, it quickly turned into anger because he never seemed to listen. He was obsessed with danger like a caricature of a Jewish mother—speaking only to give us dire warnings. It drove us crazy. When we were in our 30s, he would still tell us to look both ways before crossing the street.

"Was he ill?"

"Over the years, my therapists suggested that he may have had a personality disorder. His fears and inability to relate suggested it, but I could never find one that really fit."

"What was his occupation?" Then, before I could answer, Berry asked, "Would you close the blinds, Darling?"

The sunlight was intense. I got up and adjusted the angle to let in as much light as possible without any direct sun. Why did this give me so much satisfaction? I started talking again as I walked around the bed, returning to the chair.

"Dad was an architect. So was his older brother, but they got out of college during the depression and couldn't find work. My grandfather set them up in a package liquor store business."

"A sure thing after prohibition," Berry observed. "He must have been an astute businessman."

"He was. He was an immigrant but he quickly learned about the stock market and real estate or maybe he already knew about them in Russia. Sent his kids to college which was unusual for that generation. I guess Uncle Maury learned about stocks from him, but Dad never seemed to deal with that stuff. He worked on some architectural projects with his brother but never intentionally left the liquor store like Maury did.

"Did your parents get along?"

"Dad always showed his disappointment in Mom and I think once she saw she was never going to be appreciated, she became bitter. You know, she couldn't cook a meal just like his mother did. But she knew he was essentially a good person and she cherished the security he offered. However, she was angry all the time, trying to keep a lid on it. You could feel this undercurrent. It was very disturbing. Luckily, she had a lot of lady friends who were more like her family."

"Well, who taught you your good manners?"

This wasn't the first time Berry had brought up my manners. She seemed to sincerely enjoy them. Still, I couldn't quite believe she wasn't making fun of me.

"I guess they both had good manners. At least for the public," I answered gloomily. "They snapped at each other a lot, neither of them ever admitting to be at fault. They never apologized for harsh words, never said 'I love you' to each other or us—until Mom was dying. I told you about that."

"Your dad must have had some artistic inclinations, choosing to be an architect."

"Both of my parents did. I remember my dad writing a letter once and showing it to me. I can't imagine who he was sending it to, perhaps the local newspaper. It had a very flowery description of a sunlit day and the trees lining the street. He was taking delicious pleasure in his words. It's a strange one-time memory; he didn't write generally as far as I know."

I described how my mom was always making little craft projects, whatever fad was going on among her friends. If they were doing it, she did it, too. She sewed clothing and window treatments, made little papier maché sculptures, created pottery, embroidered, did needlepoint, assembled dried flower collages, painted scenes inspired by the variegated pattern on small slabs of marble. When she decorated her condo after my dad died, she really did a nice job choosing upholstery and carpeting for the living room, refurbishing her old furniture.

"Well, I think you should try writing about your father next."

I moaned quietly. "I don't know. At least I came to some resolution with my mother. I've spent so many years fighting the chaos of my father's fears, I can't imagine purposely going there. Afraid I'll get stuck in it."

Berry laughed, "That sounds just like the fear you told me new hypnosis clients have—afraid they'll get stuck in it." Then she sighed, "It's not that I don't understand being fearful, you saw me worry about Kathryn's driving down to New Orleans but, you know, fear is just a lack of belief. 'Anxiety is the prerequisite of sin.'"

She was quoting someone, but as I was trying to catch up to the name I'd never heard before, Rheinhold Neibor, a theologian, Berry was still talking.

"When we try to create safety where there is none, that is when we're tempted to steal, to lie. We're always looking for safety, certainly. But you have a strong fear of exploring your inner chaos. If you want to write, you'll have to. Also, it will help you be able to say something more than the words' meanings, and when you do, you'll know you can write with direction."

I hadn't thought about my fears of life affecting my ability to write. I assumed years of therapy had calmed or at least desensitized me to my turmoil. As usual, Berry had patiently waited until I was making observations about an issue before she made comments that would encourage me to look at it in more depth.

"Your dad sounds like the interesting one to write about," she concluded, "big conflicts in his personality, sensitive and affectionate, yet uncompromising, driving everyone away. A real tragedy."

Was Her Mother With Us?

*What is important about the placebo response is that
it demonstrates beyond a doubt that thoughts can trigger the
body's self-healing abilities....If we can be "tricked" into healing,
why couldn't we heal "on purpose"?*
- Martin L. Rossman, MD

I always brought my stories on paper. I liked handling the pages, making note of Berry's suggestions as well as memos on other things—books or authors she recommended, things to do, such as mailing a letter or buying food.

I hadn't looked forward to this assignment.

"There's no magic in this tale like there was in the others. I can recall only one special thing that happened with my dad. When I was very little and before knowing how to tell time, I knew exactly when he was coming home after work." Unsure I could fulfill this assignment, I added, "The mystery in the previous stories inspired me, creating an energy that insisted on my writing them."

Nevertheless, Berry asked so many questions that dozens of images of Dad were all stirred up and ready for plucking. Still, it was with reluctance that I brought the first pages.

When I finished reading them to her she said, "Now, that wasn't so bad, was it?" After I shook my head diffidently, she asked, "Would you put the breakfast tray by the sink?"

Berry was eating less and less, I noticed, only the cheese off the top of the eggs today.

Aloud, I said, "We're still in the easy part when everything was okay. But that didn't last long."

Then, pursuing a different line of thought, I said, "I spent so much time in therapy over the years returning regularly to talk about home, yet there's something different that seems to be happening as I try to write a story rather than make a journal entry. I have to enter into the time and feel it as if it's in the present just to be able to remember how the setting and the people felt to me. When I do, something actually happens—changing my emotions. I can re-experience the old feelings and also change them by bringing my present understanding to them. It's like doing Gestalt Therapy. Do you know Gestalt?"

Berry shook her head and looked expectant. I felt spoiled having her always interested in hearing some story of mine, yet it was a deep pleasure to have someone to tell about these things that meant so much to me.

"Gestalt psychology is what first made me understand the idea of experiencing an alternate reality."

Berry looked at me questioningly. I explained, "Sometimes you are asked by the therapist to act something out and even though you're just pretending, something actually happens that makes changes here in the world we all agree on—you know, the one we share by consensus, the supposedly 'objective' one. I wasn't trained in Gestalt, but I'd attended so many workshops, I grasped and was able to incorporate some of the techniques when I became a therapist. I have to tell you about this one client." Then I thought to ask Berry, "Do you want to lie flat?"

"No, but make the bed flat. I want to lean on my elbow."

I stood up to crank the bed while I talked about when I was working in a community mental health center in Chicago. Ann was a young woman who had come there for a short time about a year before. When she returned for more counseling, she became my client. Her mom, who had been the hub of their large Catholic family's emotional life, had died the year before. Since then, her father was not adjusting well to his wife's death and was depending on the kids to bolster him, but that wasn't the only challenge in Ann's life at this time. She had just recently graduated college, was unable to find a job in her field of study, had moved into her first apartment, and then her boyfriend dumped her. With all these changes and disappointments, the loss of her mom loomed to the forefront again. It was her mom who had always given comfort at difficult times and now she wasn't around to do it!

I was sitting again, saying how articulate Ann was, able to describe all that was happening yet she felt no solace from her observations. Remembering the power of Gestalt Therapy from my own experience, I asked Ann to sit in a chair and take an inventory of the difficulties she was grappling with. It's important for the patient to state everything in the present tense, helping her feel the experience again. When she was done, I asked her to move to a second chair, facing the first, where she was to act out being her mother, saying the kinds of things her sympathetic mom would have said to Ann if she could have been with her.

When Ann moved to the second chair, she began hesitantly, "Oh, Ann, I'm so sorry you're having such a difficult time." There was a long pause as she felt the recognition she gave herself with those words. With the tiniest encouragement she continued, moving more deeply into the role. "I hate to see you unhappy. You've experienced so many changes in your life in such a short amount of time." Then, silence, again, as she let that fact sink in. "Don't forget, Dear, life is always changing. You know it will get better. Just now, it seems like it'll go on like this forever."

You could see Ann's demeanor shift as she took in her mother's reminder.

"You're doing a good job," she continued. "Don't forget, I love you. I'll always be with you." Her own words silenced her. My throat tightened. Then she burst into tears and I almost did, too.

"Yes," Berry said tenderly when I finished the story. "If only we would remember." Her smiling at me caused the outer corners of her eyes to crinkle.

"On my way home that day," I said, "I couldn't stop thinking about it. How was I to interpret this session? Was Ann really contacting her mother—almost like a medium? It felt as if her mother was with us, as if another presence were in the room. The atmosphere was dense. Or did role playing allow her to own the words of comfort her mother had so often imparted in the past? Perhaps at that point Ann re-membered them, stuck them onto her own person. They truly became hers, accessible whenever she needed them. Whatever the explanation, the experience was more than a memory. Something had changed for her that day." And for me, too, I realized.

The Fifth Story—Dad

If something is too hard to do then it's just not worth doing.
You just stick that guitar in the closet next to
your short-wave radio, your karate outfit, and your unicycle,
and we'll go inside and watch TV.
- HOMER SIMPSON

I brought Berry an expanded version of the story about my dad.

Folie à Deux

It pains me to think about Dad. I'm still trying to understand how our relationship disintegrated and what the results were of my cutting him off. Of my parents, Dad was the one who had been warm and affectionate when I was little. Yet, unlike with my mother, he and I never reconciled. I was in my early thirties when he died after a long illness, still distant and unwilling to make peace.

It hadn't always been like that. When I was four, before we had a car, Dad would ride the streetcar home from work, walking almost half a mile from the stop. I so looked forward to his return that I sensed when he'd be coming and would show up at the far corner of our block just as he was approaching. Laughing over having surprised him, I also was thrilled to see his happy face grinning back at me.

Even at that time, Dad was always exhausted. He often promised but only occasionally actually walked with me to Indian Boundary Park, a special treat. I loved holding his big hand, calloused from washing glasses all day at the liquor store. About a mile to the park, two blocks along the way we passed a little cottage owned by an old lady who lived alone. Rare in the city at that time, she still had a vegetable garden with chickens and ducks walking around an unfenced yard. I admired her life. Raising animals and growing vegetables seemed magical.

At the park, we would first pass its small zoo, children's

voices carrying from the distant playground. Three or four bears in two concrete dens, a few dingoes in another. Small quarters. A distinct odor rose from the cold cement. Uncomfortable looking into their eyes, I'd sense their wildness, their prison unfair and frightening. Some deer and an array of pheasants, ducks, geese, and peacocks were together in a larger open space with bare ground. When the peacock spread his iridescent tail we were rapturous, believing we'd seen something very rare. Each spring, there were new fawns and ducklings. Sometimes I'd wonder, Why doesn't it get more crowded?

Dad would push me on the baby swings which were like high chairs with a wooden bar across the front to hold me tight, high up so Dad could push without bending over. He seemed to tire easily. Or was that just my perspective on his not wanting to push me forever? I'd go on the little slide but he and I agreed that the two higher ones and the teeter totter were too scary. His ever-increasing warnings about dangers had to be considered. The whole playground was floored with sand, making emptying socks and shoes and brushing feet carefully a tedious and necessary ritual for being able to walk home.

In the oppressive summer heat, the wading pool with a geyser-like fountain in the center called to us but I was to understand that, it, too, was not without risk. "Big" boys sat on the fountain and made the spray shoot off in unpredictable directions, causing shrieks of surprise to fill the air and prove the truth of Dad's warnings. The water must have been about a foot deep near the center, more than enough to drown in, as he explained. Eventually, the polio epidemic put an end to the pool having any standing water in it.

At the dining room table, Dad sometimes became almost playful, letting me comb his hair and pin it with bobby pins to create curls, making us both laugh. To get me to undress for bed, he'd challenge me to a race and we'd run to our rooms to change into our night clothes. I'd giggle with glee when I won. On Sundays, he religiously made a trip to the Jewish deli for smoked fish, lox, cream cheese, bagels, bialys, onion and kaiser rolls, enough bread for most of the week. Could anyone have guessed the path of this idyllic tenderness?

I always understood that Dad had been born in the old country, the city of Minsk, in the Jewish Pale Settlement. He, at five, and his brother, a year-older, came over with their mother, grandpa having arrived earlier. Aunt Lois was born here, eleven years after Dad. He was proud of being born in Russia and also of being a U.S. citizen, carrying his naturalization card with him his whole life. Whenever I asked him to tell me a story about Russia, all he would say was that he didn't remember anything about it, only that he had been seasick on the boat coming over.

Close to his parents, he talked with them on the phone almost daily. Grandpa seemed to give a lot of orders and Grandma was always sending over her special cookies. Both sets of my grandparents spoke Yiddish most of the time but they never spoke it to us, the grandchildren. Instead, all the adults used it to talk about things they didn't want us to hear.

On Sundays, Dad would buy the Tribune and read one comic to me. It was about tiny people, the Teenie Weenies. It had only one picture to illustrate it, the rest was a story, too many words for me to read. The intriguing image portrayed little people smaller than common garden flowers using both arms to lug the burden of a single walnut. A squirrel peeking at them from behind some daisies would appear monstrously threatening.

Visually, without reading the words, I was fascinated by the feeling of the different comics—whimsical Smokey Stover, the edgy chaos of the Katzenjammer Kids, the dark mystery in Little Orphan Annie, a menacing, hard world in Dick Tracy.

Dad's warnings of danger seemed to increase daily. As a toddler, they hadn't worried me. Instead, they felt like caring warmth. He was a gallant protective hero.

As we got just a little older, however, his fretting became his only response to everything, predictably dampening our enthusiasms. Little by little, thwarted attempts to talk with him became a source of growing frustration.

Still, one day, having fallen off the two-wheeler I was learning to ride, Dad told me, You're almost six now, you shouldn't cry so much. I felt ashamed. Then he took out the mercurochrome to paint the scrape on my knee. The irregular shape suggesting a face, he cleverly turned into a silhouette of an Indian wearing a feathered headdress. I gazed at my body art and my dad with admiration.

Nevertheless, it became more and more difficult to tell him about anything that happened. Good events engendered dire warnings about what could go wrong. Bad ones produced worry and reprimands. Maybe his own discomforts about what to do goaded him to tell me I was being either foolish or too sensitive. All his responses imparted the idea that I was on my own to find ways to dispatch any pesky feelings that might arise.

Every day, Dad listened to the television news and read the paper. He would repeat headlines about murder and molestations, making sure I was properly cautioned. Then he would rail against life's injustices. How could they treat blacks that way? What would make a person commit murder? Why do people fight wars? I admired what appeared to be the strength of his moral stance and his caring about the world.

At the same time, he also conveyed a deep sense of helplessness and hopelessness. On a personal level, he was unable to exert any positive influence. His unhappiness with the world, the anger that seemed to be growing between my parents, and frequent bickering among everyone in the family created an atmosphere of futility and gloom. Attempts to make him laugh were cast aside as silliness and I, too, soon felt defeated.

One day, I made a childishly cruel decision after telling Dad how Judy, a friend, had copied my drawing and how everyone was saying what a good idea she had. Her lack of crediting me hurt my feelings and I became angry with her.

You're being silly, Dad said. Copying is the best compliment a person could give you. The discussion was over. He didn't understand how much it hurt, I thought. But then, he never understood. According to him my feelings were always wrong.

I needed to show him how much it hurt. Maybe if I didn't talk to him he would ask me what was wrong and we'd be able to talk about it some more. If I already believed he couldn't respond to my just telling him he'd hurt my feelings, why did I think he was going to invite me to talk about the problem? How could I have known what this would do to our relationship?

Not talking to him was the hardest thing I had ever done. It took all of my will power. He would make some casual remark as usual and I would say nothing. Maybe he wasn't really talking to me, I told myself when he didn't seem to notice I wasn't responding. I'd just have to keep trying.

The next day it took even more will power to remain silent. To help me keep my vow, I had to stop touching him, no hugs or kisses. Determined to get him to ask me what was wrong, I persisted. Surely he'd want to know what was bothering me and then I'd be able to feel the great relief of knowing he cared and be able to tell him what had hurt my feelings.

After a third day of using every ounce of determination I could muster, he didn't seem to notice a thing. He never asked; and I never told. Less than six years old, I essentially cut off all communication, never understanding the tragedy of Dad's wounding by this terrible decision of mine.

A surprising break from our gloomy home life came when, at the age of eight, I was sent for two weeks to overnight camp along with some older children of my parents' friends. In a cabin with girls I didn't know who were my age, I cried myself to sleep the first night and on and off the next couple of days. My friend, Stef, from across the street, half a year older, was in another cabin, completely engrossed with the girls her age. Was it just the lack of familiar company that made me so sad?

We were kept busy and as I became more involved I laughed easily with all the new camaraderie, and the nickname Giggles was invented. A seasoned camper called Topper, about fourteen years old, was determined to help me through my homesickness. Attended to and loved, kept busy with nature walks, swimming, sports, and crafts, I soon felt at ease.

Allergies or a possible cold (I was always coughing or sneezing) got me moved into the half-cabin shared with the nurse's headquarters. A wall that didn't reach the ceiling divided the cabin, creating irresistible temptation. When the aliens I drew on flying saucers made from paper plates successfully landed on the nurse's side, she surprised me, soon knocking at our cabin door to play my game. I opened the door finding her beaming, saucer in hand. She wondered if we knew that Martians had been visiting her.

When the two-week camp sign-up came around, I elected to stay on, continuing to do so each time until, finally, the whole summer had passed. When parents visited, my father asked if I missed him. Torn between hurting his feelings or lying, I would skirt the issue. However, he continued to press for an answer and I admitted that I did not miss him, knowing this was the wrong way to feel. The following year I opted not to go to camp. Perhaps, if I had lied, I would not have had to deny myself the pleasures of camp. Was this to become a pattern—that everyone should have to lose?

The Rest Of His Life

And O that all would realize, come to the consciousness that
what we are—in any given experience, or time—is the combined
results of what we have done about the ideals that we have set!
- EDGAR CAYCE READING 1549-1

The story about my father continued for another twenty pages. Maybe it could have been poignant, as Berry said, but I hadn't achieved that level of writing. However, the painful exercise and talking it through with Berry did bring to me a greater appreciation of his personal tragedy and my childish attempts to reach a detente.

Berry said she was proud of my writing. I had done such a good job that all of her sympathy was with him. Knowing she meant to provoke me, I whined, "But *I* want your sympathy," and we laughed even though I meant it.

I had spoken with Berry about him many times before writing, giving her little pieces of the picture.

"He was utterly devoted to taking care of the family," I explained, "providing for us by working hard, yet everyone was at loggerheads with him. He couldn't understand emotions, and when we tried to explain, he tossed the information aside, unable to comprehend the significance of what was being said."

Another time I told her, "He heard everything only in material terms. His wife wanted to go on vacations, his son wanted his dad to take him to ball games, his daughter, well, he couldn't even figure that one out. She just wouldn't do what daughters were supposed to. She dressed like a monk with blouses that had hoods, made things with materials men were supposed to work with— concrete, clay, steel—she wouldn't get married and have children, depriving him of grandchildren. Her constant dissatisfaction kept her from seeing the obvious solutions that everyone else came up with—the tried and the true."

"It sounds like my mother's relationship with her father," Berry said quietly.

In the story, I had described several incidents of city danger and my receiving no comfort or advice because I thought I needed to protect him from seeing his ever-increasing fears confirmed.

I told Berry about his deteriorating health. He looked to modern medicine to drug or cut away the problems—satisfied that he didn't have to change anything he was doing. His decline is what first suggested to me the paradigm of holism. The many factors affecting his health were so apparent. When his dentist suggested a change of diet to address tooth loss and severe gum disease, Dad never went back to him. It was preferable to have all his teeth removed, gleefully showing off his denuded gums to everyone in proximity.

Then it was stomach ulcers. When those were *cured* with drugs, he developed colitis. The doctors suggested Dad see a psychiatrist to help reduce his anxiety. "The nerve of them!" Instead he opted for taking eighteen medications, showing them off like trophies. "Half of them are for my physical illness and the other half are to counter the side effects they cause."

Next was appendicitis. He moaned all night for days. Only when he couldn't stand up due to the pain, did he finally see the doctor who removed it. They'd never seen an appendix like his. The doctor said it was scarred from having burst several times before. Later, he had a colostomy, which was followed by infection in the abdomen caused by a glass tube left there accidently. Then a stroke. A year in rehab and another stroke, this time fatal. What a long and painful death!

I told Berry, "At one time, still during the colitis process, when he was eating an entire chocolate cake each day, someone had the temerity to suggest it might be contributing to his digestive problems."

Berry looked at me askance.

"It wasn't me! I had long given up trying to help. He had answered, 'Life isn't worth living if I can't have that simple pleasure.'"

How had it come to be that life held so little for him? I didn't know why I asked, for I had followed in his footsteps. Nothing seemed to have a meaning or purpose. I felt suicidal for years. Yet, some glimmer of hope must have kept me looking for answers.

"Had he ever had a spiritual life?" Berry asked.

"The only time I saw signs of one was when his mother died suddenly. Grandma broke her hip and the next day a blood clot travelled to her heart and killed her. He recited Kaddish at the temple every daybreak, mourning for an entire year! He had never gone to temple, not on Sabbath or even for the High Holidays."

Berry mused, "Maybe if he had gone to God for himself, he could have found some tranquility."

I thought of the dozens of small decisions I had seen him make to resist, ignore, or neglect things that were more far reaching than they appeared to him. How had this sensitive articulate man come to this?

"Before his final illness I tried to make peace with him, telling him how much I appreciated the educational opportunities he had given me. When he said nothing in response, I held his hand and continued on about the great schools I had gone to. He kept silent, a few tears rolled down his cheeks until finally he snapped, 'Well, I'm sorry I did it. You might have been better off not going to them.'"

Shaking her head, Berry said, "Determined to be unhappy. How did your mom deal with all this?"

I sighed. "Actually, the sicker he was, the easier it seemed to be for her. Without the interference of ordinary daily activities, it became much clearer what she was supposed to do. Which reminds me...on one of my trips home, I accompanied her to visit Dad in the hospital. She had been visiting him daily. This was after the first stroke. He was feeble and unbelievably thin. There was no conversation. We just sat with him; he was aware of our presence. His light blanket had worked its way down baring his chest to the waist. With great difficulty he got hold of it, awkwardly pulling it up to his chin. Mom finally took note, and with great tenderness, pulled it back down, saying, 'No, Manny, it's hot in here.'"

Berry hooted. That's why I loved talking with her. I never had to explain anything. She instantly understood how this woman with no ill intent or empathy affected her highly sensitive husband and daughter.

The frustration stirred by thinking of Dad reminded me, "You know, aside from knowing when he was going to arrive at the corner when I was little, there was one other arcane event indirectly related to him. It happened just after I made that effort to thank him for my schooling. I was listening to a tape recording of a past-life reading given to me by a Mr. Abrahamson. I had learned about him through friends in Virginia Beach. He lived in Oregon and we had agreed to a time for him to 'tune in' to me."

"What does that mean?" Berry asked.

"He suggested I meditate during our appointment hour when he would connect with me in some way. I had told him nothing about me and was living in Chicago at the time. There were a lot of enigmas contained in the tape he sent. He began with the description of a life seal with images and a word relevant to the meaning of my life. The center of the seal contained the word 'compassion' with a picture below it of live flowers growing from the ground. The background colors were an unusual combination of a deep yellow and turquoise lighter in tone than the yellow, matching a collage I had made several years before. Even now, after the passing of so much time, the color combination thrills me.

Berry pressed her hand to her head, then brought her attention back.

"Each life I was supposed to have lived had some quality that seemed very familiar about it. The one that affected me most, however, related to the fact that at the time of the appointment I was taking a lapidary class and learning from a friend who was a goldsmith how to do the finishing polish on gold jewelry. Gold looks quite rough and dull right out of the mold. Whenever we worked, she'd say to me, 'Are you sure you haven't done this before? You seem so at ease with the technique.' It was completely familiar to my touch yet I'd done nothing like it before.

"On the tape, Mr. Abrahamson said, 'The life you lived in fourteenth century England was most relevant to the one you're living now. Many of the members of your current family were your family then. They were all artists and architects. They did not approve of you. You left home to go out on your own. As a woman, this was very difficult to do and you had to do some...shall we say, compromising things in order to survive. You became a jeweler, shaping stones and working with precious metal. Years later, you went back to your father hoping to reconcile. He refused and this caused you great heartbreak.'

"When I heard those words, Berry, I burst into tears, the description of the feeling so immediate. Hadn't this just happened again? The sense of our repetitious family suffering *felt* like it had been going on for 500 years. If this wasn't a literal description of a past life, then what was it? A psychically symbolic description of what was going on at the time of the reading? It was enough to make me pray to come to some understanding during this lifetime. I don't know whether to call it a threat or inspiration to prevent our family from having to come together yet again to work it all out."

Berry reached for my hand, patting it tenderly.

What's So Funny?

Invest yourself in humor as often as possible;
find friends to laugh with.
Everyone should have at least one very funny friend,
and at least two others who love to laugh themselves silly.
- CLARISSA PINKOLA ESTES

"I don't understand it," I said to Berry on the day I'd told her about Dad reading me The Teenie Weenies. "I know I have a sense of humor when I'm talking with people. We laugh all the time at jokes I make, but I can't seem to do it in writing."

"You certainly could use a little humor in these stories. Besides, it's easy. I could hardly NOT bring it into mine. Did you notice how often I use euphemistic distortions disguised as praise?"

"Yes, but I don't know how to do that." I sounded petulant.

Raising her eyebrows, Berry suggested quietly, "You must not have that meanness in you."

I laughed as a thought flashed almost unnoticed across my mind. Wait a second. Was that a euphemistic distortion disguised as praise? "I know I have the meanness," I said. "I just haven't learned how to disguise it."

Chuckling, Berry declared, "I'll take on a challenge. Give me any sentence and I'll make it into something funny."

"Okay," I said, calling on a morose thought from my papers, "How about: 'It gave me hope that all children were going to be better than their parents—prettier, healthier, smarter. Now, I'm not sure how to assess the results.'"

Berry rolled her eyes to the ceiling as she thought for a moment. Then she said slowly, "Did all children become better than their parents—prettier, healthier, smarter? I looked around. Some must have turned out worse."

"You're good. Such a small change in the words..."

Berry beamed.

I asked, "What is it about humor that feels almost sacred? Something about the surprise inherent in a joke—an unexpected step in a sequence of thought we assume to be predictable. It makes me think of the comic Steven Wright saying, "I tried to day-dream, but my mind kept wandering."

While her eyes were still crinkled, Berry said thoughtfully, "The ability to change one's train of thought—do you think it's Divine intervention?"

We discussed so many topics in between our writing, I don't know if I've captured it. I rarely made notes about our exchanges, depending for this manuscript to be reminded only by stray phrases sporadically jotted directly on our writings or events listed on my daily calendar.

There was a book I'd read that I wanted to tell Berry about. In my excitement I presented her a lengthy synopsis of it—*Dogs* by Raymond and Lorna Coppinger.

Her response was flattering. "You're so intelligent. I've never met anyone with your intelligence. Of course, I haven't met that many."

I began laughing. Berry looked uncharacteristically stymied. "What's so funny?" she asked.

"You said you haven't met anyone with my intelligence, but, that you haven't met that many." Then Berry laughed, too.

"I meant I hadn't met that many intelligent people. I've met plenty of people. Your brilliance is a gift. It's something you're born with, so that's not to your credit."

I burst out laughing again and then so did she. I teased, "You seem to have a gift for disguising *praise*, as well as your euphemistic observations. I've been thinking. You've said a number of times how intellectual I am. I have a friend who is much more intellectual. May I introduce you to her?"

Berry agreed to meet Lynn.

I explained that when I first met her thirty years ago at Sherborne I knew her as someone who sang opera and played classical piano. Her silky blunt cut swung elegantly as she walked majestically through the halls intimidating everyone. She's become a bit more matronly now, yet studies math and astronomy just for fun, reading everything, including spy novels. Claiming strong peasant stock, she displays it in her overflowing gardens and spirited horses. She's always giving bouquets and plants to her friends. There's nothing that doesn't interest her.

"In that way she's a lot like you. She was at Claymont, too. I'll invite her over," I promised.

When Lynn came to visit, she and Berry hit it off right away. They decided that Lynn would visit on alternate days, and if I had a class, she would sometimes trade days with me, too.

Berry and Lynn talked about subjects that I never would have broached—the stock market, foreign policy, opera, Afghanistan, farming. Wasn't it good for Berry to have someone to talk with about these subjects or who would read to her, instead of a visitor who always made her work?

Berry's Alter Ego

We do not see things as they are but as the way we are.
- Jewish Proverb

Berry was into the third segment of her memoirs—from 1947 on. Many of the book reviews she had been writing in the late forties were being published in the New Orleans *Times Picayune*. Her mother was responding well to Dr. Fasting's treatments, Randolf was working for the Atlantic Refining Company finding oil deposits, and her brother Darrell was studying for the bar.

Still childless, she and Randolf considered adopting from the Catholic orphanage. They cared for a small child named Alison with whom Randolf had fallen in love.

"She was considered autistic, never spoke. We used to take her with us everywhere we went. One day she was watching a pigeon land on a nearby roof and pointing to it, said, 'Look!' We soon received a letter from the orphanage saying now that she was normal she had been adopted. Randolf was heartbroken, thinking of little Alison as his own child. We hadn't been considered as possible parents because we weren't Catholic."

Berry never said what her own feelings had been about Alison. She did explain that her return to the church happened years later.

Finally, Randolf and Berry's first child was born and Berry began to write in earnest.

"That's when I decided to tell the story of my alter ego, having existed before only in my imagination. Now I imbued her with enough life blood that I consequently won a Houghton Mifflin Fellowship."

When I was unable to find Berry's second book in the local library, she had Kathryn scour the attic for a copy of *The Mystic Adventures of Roxie Stoner*.

"I have this for you," Berry said, handing it to me the instant I walked in.

Slightly moth-eaten, the picture of a younger Berry stared challengingly from the back of the dust jacket. I drew in a breath when

I saw it. Not having known Berry in her healthy days, the woman on the book appeared to be a slightly aged Kathryn—rounded, yet having an earthy spareness that reminded me of the painting, *American Gothic*. Now that Berry was bony and brittle, she looked the way Berry described her youthful persona—sharp, peevish, deep. And the soft stark woman staring out from the picture depicted the Berry I was experiencing—attentive, intelligent, clever, patient, prayerful—not that she couldn't still sting when she wanted.

At home, I opened the book hesitantly. Never having read her writing, I was afraid it might contradict all of her vitality. But no, it didn't. It seemed, instead, near-miraculous. How did she put the reader right inside the head of the protagonist—an old colored woman describing her life in the South, and the people she encounters, with a saintly acceptance or humorous blindness to their arrogance? The language was so complex and elusive, I didn't think I could imitate its intricacy even if I had reason to try.

Next visit, I told Berry once again, "I find your use of language so unusual."

"You're not the first," she said. "When I won the fellowship for *Pursuit*, they invited me to New York to work on the final editing before publication. There were a bunch of young editors just out of college. They thought it was their job to organize all the subjects and verbs just as they'd been taught in school. Completely ruined it! They had mangled it so badly it was necessary to take the manuscript back home to work on it. Before computers, you know. I worked and worked and never could get it as good as it had been."

We shook our heads, sitting in silence. How ironic to give her a prize for writing only to have their own editors change it to sound ordinary. Berry broke the stillness with a request.

"I want to dictate a letter. There's a nurse's aide here who is applying to go to school and I told her I'd write a recommendation. Use my steno pad and write this down."

Suddenly she was in a rush, not allowing me to set up the laptop. Her tactful note described how kind and generous the aide was, knowledgeable about her duties and efficient in quietly carrying them out. Berry also commented on the woman's courteousness, displayed even during the most difficult situations, such as the ones that occur regularly in a nursing home

Under her name, Berry wanted me to include a short résumé—

Winner of the Houghton Mifflin Fellowship for Pursuit (1966) and The Mystic Adventures of Roxie Stoner (1974).
Frequent contributor to The New Yorker magazine (1966-1986)

I hung back, resistent to exposing Berry to a nursing school I thought would be cynical toward the honors she'd earned. However, I prepared the letter and mailed it later in the day.

"I have another assignment for you," she said. "Get James Joyce's *Dubliners* out of the library. When you've read a story, we'll discuss it. I'm too tired to do any more work today so you'll have to leave."

It was painful to be dismissed so abruptly. Berry didn't mind being short if that's what she needed. I knew she had stopped herself from curtness many times, alert to my easy dismay. Still, I had to soothe myself, saying that I'd have just that much more time at home for writing.

At the next visit, I set down the folder and two containers of hummus, turned down the volume on the TV, and began opening up the laptop.

Pointing to the TV, Berry said, "You can turn it off altogether. I'm celebrating—my roommate is gone. Now, you can close the door to the room." Speaking in a stage whisper, she added, giggling, "It makes the staff very curious."

Pointing to the book I was holding, she asked, "What do you have there?"

"It's *The Dubliners*," I said, shaking my head.

"Which story did you read?"

"*Evaline.* It's so depressing. Yes, he really conveys the scene, the way people are, but I'm just not interested in reading any more of them."

She was silent.

As I watched Berry, propped up on one elbow, my shoulder almost ached from her appearing so constricted. Before I could dwell on that thought any longer, she asked, "Would you please read *Evaline* aloud?"

I sat down, opening the book. After little more than a page, Berry interrupted. "Okay, you can stop reading," she said with finality. "I can hear how you hear his writing by the way you read it. It's obvious you'll never be inspired by James Joyce."

This wasn't criticism, just the observation of a teacher searching for a doorway her student could enter joyfully.

I enjoyed Berry's book, *The Mystic Adventures of Roxie Stoner*, and she told me a little bit about writing it.

"It grew out of a series of short stories that had been published in *The New Yorker*. I enjoyed the process of tying them together to create a novel. My gift for knowing how a woman like Roxie thinks comes from spending so much time with blacks who worked for us in my childhood. They have a way of thinking that's childlike..." I bristled over the stereotype until hearing the rest of her explanation "...less full of justifying, rationalizing, closer to spontaneity."

She brought *Roxie* up another time when I complained about my abundant use of the word 'I'.

"There's a way," she assured me. "I used it in *Roxie*." Eventually I learned why she couldn't describe it to me easily. "I'll show you how to do it later," she promised.

The Mystery Of Art

*Creativity is our true nature; blocks are an unnatural thwarting
of a process at once as normal and as miraculous as
the blossoming of a flower at the end of a slender green stem.*
- JULIA CAMERON

Berry's first roommate had been replaced, but when the second one left, no one new showed up. Beyond saying 'hello', I had essentially ignored them both, interested only in Berry. I didn't know if Kathryn was now paying for a private room or if something about Berry's condition warranted it. There hadn't been any drastic changes, just the steady decline I'd been observing all along.

Whenever I closed the door at Berry's request, one of the nursing home employees would inevitably open it to peek in. Berry would send up a cheery greeting! The person would always apologize as if they'd opened it quite by mistake. When it was closed behind them, Berry would laugh, never growing tired of this game.

She was curious about my education at the Art Institute. "Did you have any literature classes?"

I didn't remember any though we must have. We took our academic studies from the University of Chicago. "Because art classes were three hours long, two would fill the whole day. The academics were taught in the evening at the University's downtown campus, the style of teaching a perfect complement to creating art."

"What do you mean?" she asked.

"It was thought provoking. We read original works in whatever the subject was and then were assigned papers that required our thinking through some issue relating to them. The University's method was a potent rebuttal to all the biased and narrow textbooks that do the interpreting for the student."

"Do you think art college gave you a good education?" Berry asked. Formal schooling certainly got mixed reviews in her book—and mine.

"The art experience was really a different kind of education,"

I explained. "As with writing, you're trying to make the unseen visible. You're trying to show what is inside us more clearly, metaphorically, the way poetry can be more expressive than prose. Without expecting or intending it, I had intangible experiences with art that were unlike anything I had encountered before. Whatever theme was being examined through art would blossom. Like a child, it thrived from receiving interest and attention. But, like a seed sprouting underground, it did not benefit from an analysis of the process. Words like 'healing' or 'spirituality' came to mind for the first time in my life. This was not something we discussed in class."

Berry's expression conveyed satisfaction, as if she approved of what I was describing.

"A series of ceramic sculptures I made initiated the incidents. Each time fellow students casually commented on one, they named a different ancient culture it reminded them of. Those pieces felt like they came from a very old deep place inside, as if I could go back through thousands of years of human activity to find solid ground to stand upon.

"It hadn't been my intention. There was simply an urge to give expression to a feeling I was unable to name. Magic? Home? Longing? Roots? Nothing quite fits but my effort to find words churns up images even now. Caves with treasures, natural objects of profound beauty—rocks, shells, trees—forms of megalithic proportions, mysterious landscapes. Safety with a sense of relief, a sense of awe, as having arrived at a sacred site or discovering a place in nature that emanates an inherent power."

Berry opened her eyes and smiled at me. She had closed them as she sometimes did in my presence. Yet she was never sleeping. I could feel it. Almost unnoticeably, she lifted her chin in a gesture meaning 'keep going.'

"The result was a growing feeling of slowly being healed, of something torn being mended. Even scary images within these particular sculptures felt healing—perhaps the way a child feels comforted by talking about his nightmare. There was a sense of the eternal, of vitality, spirit. I had never needed such words until those sculptures came into being.

"The images were revelatory. As an artist I was learning something from what seemed to be a separate or larger source, even though that source was inside. By contrast, art work created through an intellectual exercise was what I'd call craftsmanship, practice in skillful handling of materials or in expressing ideas that emanated from the popular culture."

With another of our long silences, the subject was put to rest. Berry said, "I'd like to send a letter to my brother asking him whether it's true what I hear about people's estates being taken away to cover the exorbitant charges for nursing home care." What I had heard at Tri-State After-Care seemed to support that.

She dictated a short letter asking Darrell whether this 'taking' was authorized and, if so, could he point out where in the congressional record. Then she had me add, "Thank goodness the chopping of heads has been superseded by formal courtesy."

When I stood up to leave, I pointed the remote at the TV to turn it back on, there was a split screen. I thought we must have been looking at some B-grade sci-fi thriller. On the left, stood the twin towers of the World trade Center, with a plane crashing first into one, then into the other. Then each tower completely disintegrated from the top down, again first one and then the other. On the right side of the split was the Pentagon with a gaping hole in it, flaming and smoking.

I turned up the volume, only then realizing that the TV was still tuned to CNN. This was no movie. I glanced over my left shoulder to Berry who already seemed to realize what we were looking at. Too stunned to say much more than exclamations of disbelief, we bid each other good-by. I left her to contemplate the tragedy on her own and rushed home to spend the rest of the day mesmerized in front of the TV, trying to digest what was happening. For months afterward, it was as if we could hear the drone of machinery clearing wreckage all around. When I wasn't writing, reading memorial stories in the newspapers or watching them on TV was the only thing that brought a sense of relief from the pervasive agitation and gloom.

When we returned to Berry's memoirs, she described how thrilled she and Randolf were to have their first child.

"However, our son had the same milk allergy that I had as a babe, which Grandpapa had tamed. This time it was Dr. Fasting who came to the rescue. The boy had other dilemmas later—exuberant activity, loving to walk on high ledges. When we received a phone call from his kindergarten, he was ensconced atop a bust of Caesar. This was the highest point in the room and responding to their wish for him to come down, his solution would be to jump, which they couldn't allow. When I arrived, the teachers and administration made many suggestions of what was needed. I deduced and then felt offended by my conclusion that what they were actually advising was a different set of parents."

"But you don't sound like he was frustrating for *you* to deal with."

"I always thought he was special," Berry confessed. "Naturally, I love all my children but there was something about him...and he's the one I see the least." She looked like it hurt to think about. Then she shook her head as if to banish the vexing idea.

There was a certain contradiction in Berry's and my finding so much comfort in each other. From what Berry had said about her past drinking and my small exposure to her more strident qualities, I doubted I'd be visiting her if I'd known her before. Kathryn, I thought, who keeps in close touch, must be some kind of saint. Berry continued her soliloquy.

"Kathryn is the one that has probably suffered the most because of me and she's the one who is most caring." Then, in a rare show of melancholy, Berry added, "Sometimes I wonder just how much of my kids' heartaches are the direct result of my drinking."

Not wanting her to feel the burden too heavily, I took her hand saying, "Well, you know, some people claim we choose the situations we're born into. Maybe they have some lessons they intended to learn." Barry raised her eyebrows and looked into my eyes quizzically. "When I first heard that notion," I continued, "it riled me. It seemed to make me responsible for how my parents behaved. I didn't understand that the idea was to be responsible for how I behaved. Look at my brother and me. When he felt our-parents' attitude was unfair, he just went out and did what he needed to do for himself. He never got all twisted up trying to make them change, at the same time trying to get their approval like I did. He acted as though he were committed to his welfare.

"This is one of the great gifts I've gotten from the concept of reincarnation and karma, whether it's factual or not. I had to find a meaning for my suffering. Enough meaning to keep me going. Being here on the planet 'to learn lessons' was the only thing that gave me a handle to hold onto. If it weren't true, I still had some-thing in me willing to make efforts that would be beneficial to my personal development. I asked myself, What if it were valid that we choose to experience particular circumstances? Why would I have chosen mine? What have I learned that this situation was the perfect school for?"

"And what did you come up with?"

"It was clear my parents weren't intentionally hurtful. Although not wealthy, we always had a home and enough food and possessions to not be disenfranchised. I had just the right amount of physical illness to live in ordinary circumstances but was uncomfortable enough to need a different understanding of health than what the people around me practiced. My physical ill-ness frustrated my parents in their inability to find solutions, and, in the case of my mother, to bond with me as an infant. I would have to find answers myself in order to keep functioning.

"But what I really learned most about was the nature of emo-tional suffering. There was so much sensitivity in our family and plenty of suffering in Jewish history. How could I feel so much anguish during my childhood when I clearly had everything that was needed? Material comfort, extended family intact, educa-tion—all the trappings that should have been enough. If I had been lacking in any of them, I would have attributed my suffering to that lack. It's as if I came here to learn about the subtleties of emo-tional well-being, it's separateness from the material world. It's connection to attitude. I had to learn about compassion no matter how anyone's circumstances appeared on the outside, even for myself. Also, although I tried to blame my parents for our barren emotional life, ultimately, as an adult, I finally realized that I am responsible for the life I choose to live every day.

"How could there be people who have overcome diabolical cruelties such as unfair imprisonment, torture, their families being killed, and all the other terrors that can happen on earth, and not realize there must be an answer other than blame? If some of *those* people could find peace, why shouldn't the rest of us be able to?"

Berry Moves To West Virginia

The more and more each is impelled by that which is intuitive,
or the relying upon the soul force within,
the greater, the farther, the deeper, the broader,
the more constructive may be the result.
- EDGAR CAYCE READING 792-2

Berry finished the third section of her memoirs by describing the children when they were little—a second son, so docile she said she'd never met anyone like him; a little girl whom they adopted, who exulted in sharing their pioneering spirit; and then the birth of Kathryn. Berry dwelt on the extent of her drinking, telling about a time her alcoholic haze caused panic.

"One afternoon when I was going to pick up Kathryn at school, I suddenly became terrified. I couldn't remember if I'd seen her that morning. Had I actually taken her to school? She hadn't been around all day, so if I hadn't brought her to school, where was she? I drove there frantic with worry, almost bawling from relief when she exited the building with the other children."

Between Berry's drinking and writing, Randolf eventually

turned towards another woman. After the divorce, he arranged for Berry and the kids to take on his father's farm in West Virginia.

She said, "In addition to providing a home for his children, he must have figured it had the added benefit of keeping me at a good distance from him. We arrived at the property late in the day. There seemed to be so many people around that I just honked the horn."

"Oh, no! Squatters?" I asked.

Berry smiled. "The man who showed up was called Reuben, the love leader. I wrote a story for *The New Yorker* about him. He said he was the son of a prominent butcher in New York City. It was his goal to get teenagers to take on more responsibility to overthrow the United States government. To that end he pointed to a girl hanging by her feet from a tree. 'Sometimes it requires extreme measures,' he told me."

When Berry explained to him that she was the owner of the property and intended to move in, he became angry.

"Two weeks later we went to court to get him out. He had dismantled everything he could—doors and windows—and we had to search the pastures to collect them. The court ruled in our favor yet he was given another week before having to move out.

"It was around this time when I had developed my lung problem and had used the Gerson diet I told you about. Our family became more involved in farming, my second son, who still lived at home doing most of it, Kathryn cooking and taking on the housework. I wrote and sold stories while working at various jobs, none of which, due to my wandering attention, was ever kept for long.

"When Randolf put the farm in his and his third wife's name, I became upset, determined to find another place to live. While searching the newspaper want ads, I happened upon a listing for Teddy Roosevelt's summer house in New York where we moved immediately. Our new home town, however, had a number of bizarre aspects to it."

"How could you even think about moving again?"

"I had to! I was so angry with Randolf and I was afraid we'd be forced to move when it was even less convenient. In Herkimer

County, to escape the Russian revolution of 1917, one of the Russian monasteries had moved there. The monks in their black cassocks walked up and down the road in front of our house but they ignored our overtures to meet and talk with them. Finally, someone informed me they do not converse with women. I had been hoping we could call on them for help.

"Another strange aspect of the town was that everywhere we went there were identifiable mental health patients. It was at the time when those new medications had just been developed. Patients were let out from the mental wards, their behavior suddenly under control; but they were given no further services, such as help finding jobs or housing. I expected them to be pitiful, the way I saw myself, but instead found their oddities menacing.

"Curiously, only the local hospital seemed cordial to us. They had a famous chef who opened the dining room to the public. The hospital made more money from diners than from patients."

"That's refreshing," I said.

"Yes. It was exceptionally good, too. Then, when Randolf decided to transfer ownership of the farm to the children, they convinced me to sell the house and return to West Virginia. Once again, the farm was inhabited.

"This time, however, I had rented it out to a retired army officer and his young daughter. He turned out to be a deadbeat, having paid no rent for the six months he'd lived there. In a terrible humor when we arrived in the middle of the night, I shot the lock off the gate."

I'd heard that Berry was occasionally seen in her active days waving a gun around.

"My son, determined to calm me down, simply lifted the gate off its hinges and laid it to one side. I wasn't finished, however, and as we drove up, I fired another shot at the ground. The Colonel, fearing the worst, opened the front door, pointing his pistol right at us. Ignoring it, we got out of the car and entered the house. We had a friendly chat and his daughter gave us blankets so we could catch a few hours' sleep in the living room before daylight.

"In the morning, he said he had some business up at the

Pennsylvania Turnpike and would see us that evening. I asked for the rent. 'Oh, as soon as my ducks are in a row I'll pay it in a lump sum,' he promised. We all laughed, I, knowing we'd never see a penny. What I didn't know until our call to the sheriff, however, was that he was a dedicated criminal. His gang stole, then sold refrigeration vans after filing off their identification numbers. In the daylight, when he'd gone, I discovered a huge truck parked on the side of the house hidden from the road.

"My son organized our barricade for that night. When the Colonel returned, yelling to be let in, my son replied we weren't going to allow it. Surprisingly, the Colonel and his daughter simply got into their car and drove away. The next day, the sheriff came for the van. With the good care the deadbeat took of the house, our loss wasn't as bad as it could have been. He'd even refinished some of the floors. After we fixed all the neglected fences, we bought a herd of cattle."

That's where Berry ended the memoir. Nevertheless, we still had more work to do. She wanted to insert a few more tales that had come back to her.

"Read from the beginning and I'll tell you where to put the additions. Make a mark on the page and, when you print the inserts, we'll just put them into the three-ring binder."

Berry still didn't realize how easy it was to insert a paragraph into writing that was on the computer. However, rather than printing the whole thing out afresh, I proceeded as she suggested, intending to reprint it when she finished. Her first order of business was to name the memoir, *The Silly Servant*. Then, she told me several new stories.

During the time her cancerous cough was improving, she walked daily from where she worked in D.C. at a law firm to the train.

"In front of one of the big government buildings I was hit on the shoulders by two boys rushing from behind on silver bicycles. One grabbed my purse and the other some packages I was carrying. I fruitlessly began chasing them but a man close behind stopped me. 'Don't run, they'll drop it,' he said.

"He was right. Up ahead lay my empty purse and a couple of

the packages. I'd never been so distraught. Carrying much more cash than usual, still worse, was that I also had in my purse a $100,000 government bond payable to bearer. I cried all the way home while the conductor and my fellow commuters tried to comfort me. Surely this was the end of my worldly wealth.

"The police showed up at the law firm the next morning to put my sad tale on record. They explained that there'd be no way to get the cash back and that the bond, too, was considered cash.

"I had to console myself with the notion that God arranged for my misfortune. However, later in the morning, our shy office messenger came to me with an envelope addressed to *Bearer*. Inside was the bond; I could hardly believe this change of fortune. The office emissary said that the old man who delivered it thought the FBI would arrest his grandsons if they tried cashing it, and that he was very nice."

I loved the incongruity of her describing the old man as very nice. In another distressing event Berry related, "I sent a friend to pack up my office when I was too sick to continue teaching college. Another young professor there had already removed all of my books—some old, some signed first editions—telling my friend that I had given them to him."

When I expressed outrage, Berry seemed too quietly resigned to the injustice. Inside, I turned my anger on Berry for allowing him to get away with this thievery, only able to soothe myself with the thought that perhaps there was more to the story.

Berry said her grandmother had talked just a little about her father, Berry's great grandfather, who had been a minister.

"He took Grandmama riding circuit with him, teaching her Greek and Hebrew. She laughed about it, thinking it a waste of his time. Meanwhile, he had left the running of the plantation to a good overseer. If the cotton didn't get flooded out only one season in three, he'd become a millionaire from each sale. Most of the cotton was sold to the English," Berry explained.

We worked on the additions over several weeks, savoring each story, spending much of the time chatting about whatever else the stories brought to mind. Reminding me that 'Berry' was a family name, she was pretty certain that nearby Berryville, Virginia, was connected to her ancestors.

"My grandfather Berry was a prisoner of the North, held on a Union warship. We still have some of the letters he wrote from there."

According to Berry's mother there was one more Civil War-related story. "There had been a baby boy born to one of the African American women during the war. She abandoned it to run off and help the Union. He was called Uncle Willis and raised among the family children. Gentle and happy, he seemed never to need to know much about freedom. He lived with the family his whole life until his death at eighty. Mama said she made him kill a cat on a Sunday. He had warned her he couldn't do it but she insisted. Right afterward, he fell over dead."

Berry was satisfied to have finished. "I just wanted those memoirs for the kids."

"I'm sure they'll be glad to have them—your grandchildren even more so," I added, thinking to counter doubt Berry had once expressed about whether leaving memoirs was of any value.

"I'm almost ready to write the story about a nursing home, now. I've been working on it every night," she said, exuding a sense of pleasure.

"How do you remember it? If I don't write everything down, I can never recall what went through my mind."

"Oh, I go over it, again and again."

More Classes

If we fail to nourish our souls, they wither,
and without soul, life ceases to have meaning.
The creative process shrivels in the absence of
continual dialogue with the soul.
And creativity is what makes life worth living.
-MARION WOODMAN

At this time, I was still working two days a week at the library and had a few classes going for the county continuing education program and a couple of nearby colleges. The free lectures in Winchester were not leading to more classes, only endless new ideas were doing that. I fretted.

"They just keep coming," I told Berry, "always feeling as if each new one were the evolution of a single concept, but there's never enough time to explore anything in depth. It isn't satisfying but it's so driving, I can't stop. In addition, there are occasional counseling or hypnosis clients and classes I have to take to keep my license current."

Berry always listened patiently, usually saying only, "I wish you would just write."

"How do I know whether writing is what I'm supposed to be doing?" I asked, not really expecting her to answer.

"You'll know by the fact that you're writing," she answered dryly.

After creating eight different classes, one idea seemed to bring all of them together along with the heartfelt subjects Berry and I had been discussing. I called it *A Guided Tour Of Your Healing Mind.*

As with the others, Berry insisted, "We'll go over each class presentation." Then she lay back and closed her eyes to listen.

"I'm planning on passing out this chart," I explained. "On the left are eight terms naming some capacities of the mind—affirmations, contact with unknown powers, dreams, hypnosis, imagery, meditation, psychic phenomena, and spirituality. I chose those words as categories somewhat arbitrarily but also because their

191

popular use pretty much distinguishes one from another."

Berry opened her eyes again and propped herself up on her elbow. Regarding 'imagery,' she surprised me, insisting she was unable to visualize and therefore didn't see it as a category.

"But you write such clear descriptions!" I countered.

"The only visualizing I do when I think of a scene is to see the words typed on a piece of paper—doubled-spaced for easy correction."

Her example made me laugh. It was still a visual image, but certainly not the one expected. Then I explained, "My use of the word 'imagery' doesn't mean only visual pictures. It includes auditory, gustatory, kinesthetic, olfactory, and even something we can call 'knowing'." Only then would Berry agree to leave the word on the list.

She thought we should get rid of 'psychic' and combine it with 'contact with unknown powers.' Without knowing the examples in each category, she said, "Seven categories are better than eight. Seven has a more spiritual history." When we looked at the number of examples within each category, the change she suggested happened to improve the balance among them.

There were a lot of overlapping examples, partly because the words are derived from so many different concepts, religions, and cultures and partly because there simply did not always seem to be distinct differentiations. As I read her the chart in full, we questioned some words, defended our choices, argued about meanings, and added new words. This was the sort of discussion we called 'having fun'.

The newly revised chart buzzed in my head for a couple of days. At the next visit I had to talk with Berry about it some more.

"Through our discussions, I've come to realize I've been collecting those experiences throughout my life. I've made a point of sharing the stories about them with you when I rarely talk about them to anyone else. On one hand, I hold them as the most important things that ever happened to me but, on the other, I've claimed not to know what to do with them. It seems I've always chosen to set them aside, thereby allowing them no meaning nor holding any serious expectations of them. Suddenly, I'm painfully aware this has been neither uplifting nor helpful for putting my ideals into practice. Living that way hasn't been fun and certainly hasn't contributed to inner peace.

"Meanwhile, the experiences themselves were just the opposite," I continued, "always accompanied by a feeling of excitement. They filled me with hope, and, what may be most important, a sense of being connected to something larger than my personal world."

After having presented several of the classes, I brought up the topic of the healing mind to Berry once again.

"I've only just begun the process of changing my expectations, not finding it easy to do. I've decided to accept the mysterious experiences as they are, giving them no dismissive interpretation, instead, strengthening my understanding while educating myself to interpretations others have made about similar happenings."

Berry was still listening, not saying anything.

I added, "As I've begun sharing some of the stories in class, I'm discovering that almost everyone has had some inexplicable experience. They're also unsure of how to integrate them into their ordinary lives. Even the people who don't think they have any, after some thought and listening to others' stories, recall something. I'm hoping that by telling our stories about these gifts of the moment, we'll fortify our inklings and yearnings. I'm convinced now that these events are the sounds of our souls trying to lure us back to life."

Berry had been looking into my eyes the entire time, alert to my increasing enthusiasm.

"All we need to uncover them," I said, "is to pay attention. When we do, the first thing we discover is that they seem to happen more often than we suppose. When we receive a call from a friend just after thinking about that person, we have a strong feeling that it is not merely coincidence. Sometimes the event feels sacred even though it's related to ordinary sorts of activities. Why would it feel sacred?"

Berry was smiling at me, the outer corners of her eyes crinkling in their familiar way.

"Good," she said. "You're onto something—a way to understand all the experiences and studies you've made. You have to find a way to express it. You have so much to share."

What a kind thing for her to say.

"You seem to be the only one who believes that. I don't know what I would do without your encouragement."

Berry's Nursing Home Story

To be what we are,
and to become what we are capable of becoming,
is the only end of life.
- ROBERT LOUIS STEVENSON

Each project I worked on made me think my focus would soon become more centered. However, before long another new venture soon demanded my attention. As a licensed social worker and writer on alternative healing, I wanted to offer services to people who were drawn to alternative health care but who felt they needed guidance in making decisions, so I designed a website to that end.

It was fun trying to explain how websites worked to Berry who had never seen one.

"Imagine you open a book and look at the Table of Contents. You move a cursor to where it says 'Chapter 3' and click on it. Chapter three pops onto the screen! No pages to turn. You're just suddenly there."

"Amazing! Is it hard to create?"

"Well, I have to learn how to use the program. I used to know how and then I forgot and I can't understand the instructions manual. That's why I was going to pay someone to do it. But the artist I consulted wants $3000 for the basic design. I've just got to figure it out."

Eventually I did. Then Berry and I spent weeks going over the material I put on it. At the same time, I was teaching classes and still volunteering for the networking group and the Healing Arts Council. I was the busiest mostly unemployed person either of us knew.

Although Berry was interested in my take on alternative health care, she still expressed flashes of despair over my unwillingness to focus on writing.

"I wish you would just write," she reiterated.

"Me, too. But how am I supposed to make a living?" Silently I reprimanded myself. Would I be coming to the nursing home three times a week and writing most of the afternoon if I were really worried? It wasn't worry as much as it was logic...and guilt. Shouldn't I be working? Instead, I wanted to be with Berry, learning how to write. The societal answer was that I was being immature and irresponsible. I knew what words to call it. What would I be doing without my husband Bruce? Surely one of these things I was trying to create was going to work, wasn't it?

"I did the same thing." Berry mused. "Got so involved with earning money from the farm that I stopped writing altogether. I've felt an unexpected great happiness being in the nursing home because all the burdens of life have been lifted from my shoulders. I'm left only with prayer. And there's really only one we need. 'Thy will be done.'"

We smiled at each other. "Wouldn't that be a relief?" I asked, both of us nodding wistfully.

I cleared my throat. "Well, now we have the opportunity for you to write again, too, with no pressure to sell." I urged her to start her nursing home story, especially since she reported working on it every night. She was ready.

It was just as it had been with the memoir. She spoke slowly, looking up at the ceiling as if prudently reading some manuscript floating in the air.

Here's the gist of the story. It's September 11th and a 79-year-old Virginia gentleman is speaking, complaining about his swollen ankles. He's standing at his grandson's eighteenth birthday party, admiring for what seems to be hours, the boy's extravagant gifts. The old man can't understand why no one has thought to bring him a chair.

Already, Berry made me laugh. Her main character, Andrew J. Bultman, a retired banker, expects others to know when his ankles are swelling. As the story proceeds, he receives a phone call that day from his eighty-five year old Aunt Carrie, who lives in New York City. It's the afternoon following the destruction on 9/11 and she has decided she must come to live with him in Virginia. In the same self-centered way, she expects Bultman to pick her up in New York the next morning but he talks her into taking a train to D.C. where he and his butler will meet her.

I liked the three characters—a retired widowed businessman used to having his own way, Aunt Carrie who has specialized in writing about and preserving groundhogs, and the omnipresent butler who runs interference on all of Bultman's dilemmas.

At first, Bultman is upset by Aunt Carrie's new demands in his life. However, he reminds himself of her importance, famous for founding a missionary colony in the Far East to stamp out Buddhism.

"I don't think I give readers enough credit," I said to Berry.
"What do you mean?"
"I just assume there's so many people who believe in things like stamping out Buddhism that they wouldn't get the joke." She smiled at me and continued her dictation. I looked forward to hearing more as much as if I had been reading it in a book.

Aunt Carrie feels that the forced change in her life caused by the tragedy is Divine Intervention giving her the opportunity to save the country from destruction. Just when I was wondering how a nursing home was going to fit into the plot, Bultman suggests that his aunt stay at one, not far from his home, until he can remodel his house to accommodate her. When Aunt Carrie is angered by the home's testing her mental faculties during admission, he reassures her by reminding her how many clients they have from West Virginia.

After she is settled in, Bultman stops at a French restaurant to bring a special treat to her. She so savors the high priced prizes that she wants the food catered on a daily basis.

To complete this section, I was assigned to research the local faux French bed and breakfast for menu inspiration. We chose "Petit Canard Et Foie Gras Amiable and 'Le Perch' À La Brochette D'Asperges Et De Homard," both of us only guessing what they might be.

When I was getting ready to leave, Berry asked, "Since you weren't inspired by James Joyce, who would you be inspired by?"

Berry's Nursing Home Story—Aunt Carrie

The genius of you Americans is that you never
make clear-cut stupid moves, only complicated stupid moves
which make us wonder at the possibility that
there may be something to them which we are missing.
- Gamal Abdel Nasser

To answer Berry's question, I had to stop gathering my belongings and think hard, finally remembering a couple of writers. "I like Robertson Davies and Barbara Kingsolver for subject matter and writing style."

"I'm not familiar with Kingsolver. Is she new?"

Surprised Berry didn't know her name, I blurted out, "*The Bean Trees? Pigs in Heaven? Animal Dreams?*"

"No," Berry said shaking her head. "I'm not familiar with any of them."

I reminded myself that Berry had been sick for quite a few years and seemed to be a classicist.

"Kingsolver and Davies are probably the only fiction authors whose other books I've searched out after reading one. I read popular fiction periodically but I just don't think to look for everything that person has done. Actually, fiction doesn't draw me, especially short stories which I find exceptionally unsatisfying."

"Now, why is that?"

"They never seem to have endings...satisfying conclusions."

"Well, what kind of books do you like?" she asked.

"Memoirs. It can be by someone unknown if it's good writing. I've read quite a few poorly written ones just because they were by famous people I was curious about. I read a lot of alternative health like *Vibrational Medicine* or *The Field*, but not especially for the writing. Recently I read a couple of autobiographical books by the woman who used to be the LA Times Food writer." I had to pause again, trying to think of her name. "Ruth. Ruth Reichl! *Tender at the Bone* and *Comfort Me with Apples*. Those were great! Fun stories, well written. Or how about *Bird by Bird*, Anne Lamott? I've also read a lot of books just because of the unique subject matter. Some are well written. I'll bring a couple."

"Bring Kingsolver. I want to see what you like."

I had finished closing up the laptop. Then I put on my coat, picked up the PC along with the manila folders, and was already at the door when I turned around. "I'll see you on Saturday," I said, blowing her a kiss.

Berry threw me a kiss back with her long fingers and called out, "You can leave the door open."

When Berry continued dictation at the next visit, she had Aunt Carrie go from room to room in the nursing home interviewing patients concerning abuses to their autonomy. Bultman intervenes, fearful of her getting them into a lawsuit. Hoping to further modify her activities, he convinces an old prep school buddy, a doctor, to prescribe her a tranquilizer. When the nursing home insists on filling all prescriptions themselves, Bultman takes Carrie's rejected medications home for his own use.

My laughter caused Berry to grouse, ignoring what I was

laughing about. "It's true. Another way for nursing homes to make more money."

On Bultman's next visit he discovers Auntie has miraculously come across a lady who shared Auntie's interest in groundhogs—had even dined on them—and was an encyclopedia of knowledge. Aunt Carrie discovers the woman has a perfectly good house where she could live if only someone would stay with her. Carrie decides the two of them will go to the house to raise groundhogs for sustenance as the lady's family had done in the past.

Berry and I lived where groundhogs were as numerous as squirrels, but who would have thought of raising them for food?

She interrupted her story, fixing me with another assignment. "I want you to get a one-paragraph description of the groundhog from the library. See if you can add a little humor. This is supposed to be something Bultman reads in Aunt Carrie's book about them, published years before, copies he rediscovers in his attic."

At the library, some references listed the animal as a wood-chuck, some by groundhog, and some by *Marmota Monax*. Many didn't have any description of the animal's behavior, only its phys-ical attributes. Finally, the dependable *Encyclopedia Britannica*, where perhaps I should have looked first, provided a solid struc-ture to work from.

Berry explained that slipping in some well-thought out adjec-tives was all that was needed for humor. "Use words that aren't quite right for the meaning of the sentence," she said. I was so excited to have a method spelled out that I got over-enthusiastic and Berry had to cull a few of them out.

In the assigned paragraph, I admired the groundhog for gain-ing fat to survive its winter nap. I called hunters unscrupulous for shooting the animal when it displayed its unfortunate habit of standing tall and accused farmers of being unfeeling for consider-ing groundhogs pests for eating their crops.

"Yes," said Berry, "You're learning to distort things nicely." I'd never been complimented for *that* before.

The ending, a fact summarized right from the encyclopedia, got a bigger laugh from her than my intentional efforts. It described the paradox of Groundhog Day when good weather serves as a bad omen foretelling six more weeks of winter.

Berry invited me to join her in considering the name of Aunt Carrie's new companion. Eula and Wanda were my nominations but Berry settled on her own contender, Wilma.

Bultman arranges for his ancient butler and the butler's wife to go down to Wilma's farm with the ladies to get them settled in. When the butler phones to report, instead of hearing a failed scheme as Bultman is expecting, they sound energized and years younger.

Now that they were out of the nursing home, how would Berry ever return to the topic? My musings were cut short.

"That's all I want to do today. Would you please put the blinds down?" Berry asked.

I stood up and walked around the bed. "Do you want the window closed, too?" The aide had opened it to let in some fresh air. I had arrived when Berry was being changed. She nodded. I shook the cord to lower the blinds and then adjusted them. It was still early in the visit, so I let her know, "I brought one of Kingsolver's books."

"Good. Let's hear it." I hadn't read but a paragraph before she stopped me. "I don't like it. I don't want to hear any more."

"What don't you like?" I was disappointed.

"She's just too cutesy. I can't stand that casual humor, like she's your buddy..."

"That's just what I like in this one." Not totally surprised by Berry's dismissal, however, I put the book away. Maybe I should have brought later Kingsolver's like *Prodigal Summer* or that missionary one set in Africa—*The Poisonwood Bible*. No, I doubted Berry would like any of my choices in fiction. Our tastes were so different.

At the next installment of Bultman's tale, Berry has him receive a call from Aunt Carrie who's still down at the farm. She's in touch with a producer of documentary movies interested in the groundhog story. During Berry's dictation I had an internal running commentary: A documentary! How did she think of that?

To Aunt Carrie's joy, the producer has caught on to her idea—

a meat shortage caused by mad cow disease, not enough hogs to fill the need. Groundhogs. The perfect solution.

Bultman interrupts her exposition of the grand concept with, 'How are you doing, Dear?'

I loved that Berry has him intrude to say something so circumvent, again insinuating so much about his personality. Once she named the technique—elliptical—I was better able to recognize it. But, still, I bemoaned her not writing about a nursing home. The story had wandered far afield, I thought.

Auntie needs money to invest in the filming. Bultman maneuvers their combined fortunes in the bank, ostensibly to protect hers from the 'Hollywood robber', while raising doubt in the reader's mind about his own honesty—another layer of thought that drew me in.

Berry's Nursing Home Story—The Idealist

Do not be critics, you people, I beg you.
I was a critic and I wish I could take it all back because
it came from a smelly and ignorant place in me
and spoke with a voice that was all rage and envy.
Do not dismiss a book until you have written one,
and do not dismiss a movie until you have made one,
and do not dismiss a person until you have met them.
It is a ****load of work to be open-minded and generous
and understanding and forgiving and accepting, but,
Christ, that is what matters. What matters is saying yes.
- DAVE EGGERS

Berry smiled as she described Bultman's ruminating. Though Carrie is neither sick nor dead, he is thinking about her funeral. He gets stuck on what to put on her tombstone. 'Carrie Livermore

Bultman, 1916-20__. Patriot, Lover of Wildlife.' He concludes that it is too banal, settling instead on 'An Idealist.'

This became the title of Berry's story.

The documentary movie maker rejects the possibility of Auntie writing the script because her style is too scientific. I laughed at that and then again as Aunt Carrie says, 'the producers want romance.'

In the meantime, Bultman's daughter-in-law wants her son, Andrew III, a senior in high school and the original birthday boy, to play the leading man. In an additional complication, Auntie has determined to adopt her companion Wilma's niece, Violet. Andrew III and Violet spend time together at the groundhog farm. The ladies' raising chickens is added to the mix, water pumps are installed, a plumber is brought to the farm, turkeys are hunted, and groundhogs trapped to establish the new industry. Everyone involved is phoning Bultman with the latest news which he doesn't really want to hear.

Berry hadn't been feeling well the last couple of visits. "Are you up for working today?" I asked as I took off my coat and hung it on the back of the chair.

She nodded. "Just a little. I'm doing better today."

As she leaned back, I helped push the black pillow in place and then turned off the TV.

When the computer was set up, Berry asked, "Where did we leave off?"

I opened the manila folder, reading the last page. "The daughter-in-law was phoning in her report to Bultman."

"Oh yes." Berry had the daughter-in-law complain about Aunt Carrie going berserk with her lofty plans.

All the phone calls convince Bultman he needs to go down there with the butler, of course, and give Auntie a good talking-to. When he does, she counters, telling him that rehabilitating young people is the most important work she has ever done along with starting a thrifty American business. Furthermore, she characterizes Violet as a sensitive and trusting young girl. I enjoyed the surprise of Violet being portrayed sympathetically.

During the visit to his aunt, Bultman awakens in a hospital room with his butler at his side, who explains to the old man that he has been unconscious for three days, but that he'll have good company when he gets home as Violet and Andrew eloped and plan on living in his house to take care of him.

The ending was sudden and funny. However, I was still disappointed Berry hadn't given nursing homes a good going-over.

She had me send off the story to *The New Yorker* with a cover letter stating her inability to read or write and her intention to dictate a series of stories about the fun we have in West Virginia.

I said to Berry, "I'll include a photocopy of the dust jacket of *Roxie Stoner* because the fly leaf mentions that most of the stories from *Roxie* were published in *The New Yorker*."

To my surprise, the following week, Berry insisted on making a significant addition to *The Idealist*.

"But we already mailed it," I protested.

Unruffled, she said, "We'll just have to send them the revised version."

In the continuation, Bultman's son, Andrew II, has Auntie and Wilma certified by a psychiatrist and conveyed back to the nursing home. Andrew III, now Violet's new husband, is sent back by his father to finish high school. Meanwhile, Bultman befriends Violet who is now staying at his house. He is utterly charmed by her, determining she must finish school and remain living at his place to help care for Auntie at the nearby nursing home.

I thought I could see where the story was going, that romance would blossom between the old man and the girl. I became impatient, thinking it would require too much manipulating to get everything resolved. The next few sessions Berry was having a bad spell again but she continued the narrative—a little more slowly than before.

Bultman and Violet's lunches together are disturbed only by her apparent digestive problem. He has the butler take Violet to the doctor, his prep school buddy. She returns blushing with a note written on a prescription pad, saying, 'Congratulations!'

Bultman tells his son, Andrew II, that Andrew III must marry her. His son reminds him that Andrew III and Violet already are married. Bultman orders him to get Auntie out of the nursing home and give her the front bedroom and bath.

I was taken aback. This wasn't at all where I thought it was going. Bultman ludicrously claims to finally be himself—decisive and commanding. He plans which rooms everyone will live in, designating the front parlor his own and congratulating himself. He had borne the responsibility for four generations of his family and prayed to live to see the fifth. He begins to ruminate about his own tombstone and comes up with:

'And how can man die better
than facing fearful odds,
for the ashes of his fathers
and the temples of his Gods?'*
* Thomas Babington Macaulay 1800-1859 (American)

Suddenly, the story was over. I laughed with delight, realizing that just when it felt as if the narrative would become tedious, Berry resolved it in a totally unexpected way.

She was pleased with my reaction. "Print a copy and send it to *The New Yorker*," dictating another cover letter explaining the revision. A few weeks passed before we heard anything.

The New Yorker sent a form rejection letter and didn't even return the manuscript. I thought it unkind and Berry did not hide a look of keen disappointment. Two days later, however, a large envelope arrived. In it was the manuscript and a personal letter from the editor. *The Idealist* was still rejected but at least Bill Buford was personally cordial.

He wrote: "We all enjoyed reading it—it's engaging and funny and elegantly done. But we didn't think it would work out here. We do hope you find a good home for it, though. Thank you for letting us see it. And we'd be glad to read more."

Berry and I sent *The Idealist* to two other magazines which also rejected it. I had wanted so much for her to have one last sign of recognition from the professional outer world.

Another Writing Assignment

Hope
It is not 'Have I got a chance?'
It is more often: 'Have I seen my chance?'
- IDRIES SHAH

Putting aside the notion of doing any more writing, Berry said, "I think it's time for you to tackle a story about your mother."

Although Mom and I had come to a delicate resolution in our relationship, I felt almost paralyzed confronted with writing about her. Berry and I had both discussed our mothers quite a bit by this time yet Berry had to walk me through the first few pages, the same as when I couldn't figure out how to expand my earliest vignettes. Again, she created sentences for me, one by one, from my descriptions. Then I would rewrite them to more precisely portray the experience.

She also showed me how to write from inside the little girl's head so I wouldn't have to use 'I' so often. This was the technique from *Roxie* she had promised to show me. It took a while to get the hang of it.

She said, "The way I described it to my students was to have them initially write their story in the first person. It helps you remember details, then tell the same story in the third person. You can use the third person even when you are in the head of the person telling the story."

I couldn't understand what that meant until we tried it. I used a different name for myself as the child, Berry thinking this might give me some emotional distance. As many times as I had described my childhood in therapy, the exercise of writing it using Berry's techniques resulted in a different emotion. There was no longer a sense of blame or defense.

However, for three visits the writing inched along with Berry pulling each sentence out of me as if she were hauling a rock-loaded bucket up from the bottom of a cliff. I was awed by her patience. One day, finally, I went home and wrote several pages by myself, ecstatic over the breakthrough.

After reading the first few pages to her for the fifth time another day, I asked Berry, "Isn't this tedious for you?"

"I live for this," she answered tenderly. "You should be the one who's bored, my making you read it again and again. You're such a good student."

"I'm not bored at all; I feel lucky. Amazed by the process. Changing a word here, another there, and then the whole feeling shifts. What has astounded me throughout our months together is when sometimes you make up something, telling me that circumstances like that must have happened in order for the story to proceed as I've indicated and, sure enough, I remember something—not actually the same exact event you suggest—but something that supplies the same motivation. It's uncanny."

"I can't die until we get you published," Berry stated with finality.

How sweet! But I said, "Kind of puts me in a double bind. I'd love to get published but I don't want you to die."

"Well, we don't actually have that choice. Anyway, thanks to you, I've been having all this fun. I never expected it at this stage of my life."

"Me neither. In fact, we've had so much fun writing together, I wonder if I'll even want to write without you."

"Oh, you will," she assured me.

At the library where I was still working, I had learned from Brenda that shoestring potatoes, which I mentioned in my story, were still sold, still packed in a soup-size can. When I brought a can to Berry to celebrate my writing breakthrough, I was saddened by having forgotten that Berry couldn't chew such crunchy food.

"You'll have to feast on those by yourself," she said curtly, and then reading the disappointment on my face, spoke more softly, "That's okay. You enjoy them. I'll join you with hummus."

I certainly didn't need help polishing them off while reading the next section to Berry. How in the world had four of us at home shared one little can?

There was a rumor at the library that the board thought that if Colette and I continued sharing her job, the library could pay less wages for our part-time work. Suddenly Collette was never available when I phoned her. Did she think I had been trying to arrange it so she couldn't come back full time?

I loved the job but had understood it was temporary. Berry warned me, "Behave in a civilized manner no matter what happens." I willingly took her advice. Something in me had softened. Was it the result of having Berry so thoroughly on my side?

At the end of the week, the director tearfully told me that Colette was returning and that this would be my last day. I phoned Bruce who happened to be working at home that day and asked him to bring donuts for everyone at around three o'clock. I decided to surprise them by giving myself a going away party. To complete my assignment, I phoned Colette the next day, thanking her for job-sharing and wishing her well. I hoped our pleasant chat conveyed that I hadn't been trying to do any harm.

Worry

What one thinks continually, they become;
what one cherishes in their heart and mind they make a part of
the pulsation of their heart, through their own blood cells, and
build in their own physical, that which its spirit and soul must
feed upon, and that with which it will be possessed, when it
passes into the realm for which the other experiences of
what it has gained here in the physical plane, must be used.
- EDGAR CAYCE READING 3744-5

Berry, becoming weaker, was now barely able to feed herself.

"My contract with the nursing home states that they can't feed me," she reiterated. After a long pause she asked, "Do you know how long it would take to die from starvation? Not that I could hurry death along yet because everything still tastes so good."

To answer Berry's question, I brought her the skillfully-written, *Dying Well: The Prospect for Growth at the End of Life* by Ira Byock, M.D. Byock was director of a hospice in Montana and past president of the National Hospice and Palliative Care Organization.

While searching the index, I said, "Nothing on starvation, maybe there's a euphemism. Here it is, 'Eating, stopping of' and 'Food, lack of, refusal of, and withholding of'."

Byock introduced the topic through the story of a patient whose terminal illness caused him to choke when eating. Afraid he would die choking, he asked the doctor if starving would be a painful way to die. The doctor explained that it wasn't. Deciding whether to stop eating or to continue feeding himself or be fed through a tube were entirely up to him. This was one area of his life where he still had control.

The doctor also made a different point by asking him how his appetite was.

"I lost it long ago," he answered. "Eating is just habit or I do it to please my son." Being clearer about his current relationship to food, his next question was how long death would take.

Byock told him, "It's always hard to say how long someone is going to live, even in this situation. I don't think it would be long, perhaps two or three weeks. Probably less if you stop taking in fluids....People usually become increasingly sleepy and gradually drift away peacefully, without any pain or other discomfort."

In Byock's book, when the family of another dying patient said they did not want the patient to die of starvation, Byock posed the question: What would be acceptable for her to die of? He told them that at the end of a long illness people often stop eating, that it is the wisdom of the body and one of the more peaceful ways to die.

Berry heard enough. "You can stop reading now. Thank you. I want to add just one more section to my memoirs, a little history about relatives I hadn't actually met but know something about."

She didn't remember that we had already written most of those stories but I said nothing. I didn't mind hearing them again and Berry seemed content.

I was thinking about Byock's book. Berry's situation wasn't exactly comparable to the examples he gave about not eating. She was experiencing a lot of pain and it was increasing. Byock had also discussed using palliative drugs carefully so that pain would be controlled without putting the patient into a stupor. It required an attentive and knowledgeable staff to come up with the right mix.

Berry interrupted my thoughts. "Let's read the next section of your story."

"What did your mom tell you about your birth?" Berry asked during another visit. I remembered mentioning it in one of the earlier versions of the story, but it wasn't in the one I was reading.

"She must have been scared," I answered. Then suddenly remembering something Mom had said about her pregnancy, I told Berry that account first. "Dad had his heart so set on having a girl this time that Mom worried constantly about what she would do if the baby turned out to be a boy."

"Another part of your Dad's tragedy," Berry suggested, "getting what he wanted and it still didn't work out."

We both sighed. "The reason I assume she was scared at the actual delivery was because of this anecdote she told many times: They arrived at the hospital before midnight and apparently her contractions were so strong she was afraid she'd give birth before the doctor arrived. She said she did everything she could to hold me back. I always wondered if that hadn't set the tone of our relationship."

It wasn't until I had neared writing the end of the story about Mom that we worked on the name. Our dialogue led naturally to my focus on the feeling of isolation, eventually leading to *The Wall*. It was Berry who refined it to *Walls*.

When Berry and I were done looking at the final section, I said, "My friend Tara told me last week that she had a dream about my mother. It startled me because I'd been having a feeling at odd moments over a week's time that Mom was looking over my shoulder and trying to get my attention. I purposely ignored it, feeling guilty about not painting all that nice a picture of her."

"What was the dream?" Berry asked. She was lying back, the bed flat, as it was most of the time now. The amount of food stains on her top revealed the increased difficulty she was having feeding herself.

"Tara was at a party and my mother came right over to where Tara stood saying she wanted her to give me a message. Trouble was that Tara couldn't remember it when she woke up. We had laughed over it. I think I was relieved. Well, a few days later, when Tara was at my house again, she told me, 'I had the party dream again! Your mom must be determined.'

"This time Tara remembered a series of uncharacteristically heartening little comments Mom wanted her to pass along ending with, 'Tell her I want her to find peace. That is the most important thing—find peace.'"

Repeating her words aloud, I had to blink away tears. "It's not typical of Tara to pass along messages from the dead."

In another of Berry's infrequent moments of physical tenderness, she took my hand, "Maybe now your mother understands more than she used to."

Completed, the story about Mom wasn't as long as Dad's had become and it held together better. "I've learned a lot from writing this one—including your *Roxie* technique of being in the character's head," I said slowly.

"So what's the hesitation I hear in your voice?"

"Oh, I think it's a good story, but it's not the kind I would seek out to read. I'm also finally understanding the idea of saying something without spelling everything out in that expositional way I tend to fall into."

"Yes. We did manage that." Then Berry leaned back. "Read it through again." I watched her face relax as she closed her eyes to listen.

The Sixth Story—Walls

An atheist is a man who has no invisible means of support.
- JOHN BUCHAN

Walls

The mother never raised her voice. You're always asking for something, she said to her little girl. I just now sat down to read the Tribune. I'm a week behind.

What could she ask, Lily wondered? When you were little, could you cross the street by yourself?

I used to go to the store for my mother.

It had worked.

The store keeper admired my Yiddish. What will it be, young lady? How was the smoked fish last week?

But, did you cross the street by yourself?

A deep sigh. There was no street to cross. The store was on the corner of our block.

Oh, well. When would it be safe to talk again, when she was turning a page? But Mom had already turned away, her profile set against the window.

Go play with your dolls, Lily.

This just meant the dolls you could touch. Upstairs in her room these dolls lay on a toy bunk bed. All you could do with them was take their clothes off and put them back on again. Then what? Up on the wall, the storybook dolls were arranged in rows in their boxes, their lashed eyes peeping out through the shiny cellophane. What did they see? Did they want to come down and play? That would be out of the question. How could you get them back up again? Mother said you can't play with things that are on display. And when people came, they always admired these the most. Who came? Her cousins. A new lady friend came once, holding an infant baby. Her mom was showing the dolls to her when the baby began fussing.

211

Mom cooed at it and it stopped crying.

Babies and puppies always love me, she said. Then she turned to Lily suddenly. You're jealous, aren't you? Was she supposed to answer? A new girl and her mother came once, too.

Maybe in the closet there would be something new to see. There was the dress Mom had picked out. It itched at the waist but there wasn't anything to do about it. She knew all the shoes. Behind the clothes, only another wall. No door. But wait, there was the brown cardboard box with her soda fountain dishes. Miniatures of real life sundae cups and banana split dishes. Each piece stacked with it's own kind and fitted into a cardboard holder. She loved them. She took them out one time and couldn't squeeze them back in.

Don't take things out if you can't put them away properly.

So, what to do now? Downstairs, again, looking out the front screen door, the little girl across the street had gone inside. Mother was still at the dining room table reading.

I didn't know Judge Goldberg died, she said. What of? It doesn't say.

Was it time for lunch? In the kitchen was the bread drawer you could look into. Full of bread and cupcakes. It usually had some challah and today there were her favorite chocolate-covered marshmallow cookies.

What are you doing?

Mother must have heard the sound of the drawer being opened.

I was hungry.

Don't eat any cookies.

Oh, well, it would soon be time for lunch—maybe bananas and sour cream.

Dad was coming into the house now. He was carrying a bag. That's right, this week he didn't have to work at the liquor store until later.

You'll ruin your appetite.

He must have heard what Mom said. But, after lunch, he'd

help her get the milk down by letting her have as many cookies as she needed.

He turned around and went back to the front door. But it was only to put his coat and brimmed hat into the closet. He said he had been out to the bank and the bakery. Now, he kissed the top of her head. What had he brought? Dad took out the salami that hung in the kitchen closet and made himself a pumpernickel sandwich, cutting a nice chunk of salami for her.

Mom came in and took cottage cheese from the Frigidaire.

At mealtime, they didn't talk. They used to listen to the radio. That was when they ate in the little breakfast room off the kitchen. Now, with the TV in the dining room, they all sat around one side of the table so you could watch. At lunch time, on TV, Uncle Johnny Coons showed silent films. Daddy and she loved that—Charlie Chaplin and the Keystone Cops. Sometimes Buster Keaton. If Dad was home at night, they would watch Ozzie and Harriet or Father Knows Best with Robert Young. Those parents always talked to their kids.

Why didn't you tell me Judge Goldberg died? Mom asked.

I mentioned he was very sick a couple of weeks ago.

Yeah, but now he's dead.

Without saying anything more, Father went back to watching Charlie Chaplin. Should she ask who Judge Goldberg was but, no, they already looked upset.

Suddenly wanting to leave the room, Lily picked up her glass quickly and splashed milk on the pink plastic table cover. Father snapped, Why'd you do that? When her mom clucked over the spill, Dad seemed to be waiting for her to make a move, then, stomped out to the kitchen sink to get the dish rag. Didn't Mom see she was supposed to get it? But when Dad got angry, you couldn't feel sorry for him.

Where could she go to get away from this? No place in the house. In the back yard? Dad said, Okay, but don't leave our yard. The house was never left unlocked. She would have to ring the bell to get back in.

The yard was quiet. The brats next door were in school. Her brother Neal was, too. She walked to the empty concrete pond at the far end and sat on the edge with her feet inside. It was rectangular, about a foot deep. Daddy said it had been a fish pond. There was a drain at the bottom, but never any water. The big cracks must have let it leak out.

It would be nice to have your own cabin on this spot. Just her size, like the lady with the ducks and chickens they saw on the way to the park. Living all alone or only with brave Hopalong Cassidy. She'd feed the wild birds and they would land on her arms when she held them out. Birds you didn't have to be afraid of. They would fly away if you looked at them too hard. They'd sing on the roof and build nests in the corners of the windows. They didn't seem to need anything but gentleness.

Maybe Hopalong would teach her to hammer together wood to make walls and use the pond for the floor, but how could you make the wood stick to the concrete? Oh well, Mom and Dad would never let her live there anyway.

On one side was the little pine tree—a bit taller than she was. On the other side a flowering tree. Last year it was like a pink cloud on her brother's birthday. Each flower like a tiny rose.

Behind her cabin would be those same hollyhocks standing like soldiers next to the garage, but some too far apart and some too close together. She'd have to fix that. To the side of the garage, by the door, you had to walk under an arch of sweet smelling white blossoms. Along the rest of the way to the alley were those violet colored flowers—a drop of honey to suck from each one when you pulled it off the stem. The other side of the garage was wild, too shaded for grass but full of plants, anyway, and rocks. Even a vine on the fence! A bird apartment house sat way up on a pole. Over there you could find rocks the size of baking potatoes near the garage—big smooth ones and little jagged ones, sometimes with imprints of sea shells on them.

The smooth ones were heavy, made up of sparkly silver, black, and colored specks. So pretty. You could scrub them clean. Now, when mother opened the door she lugged three of them into the house.

Why are you bringing those in?

I'm going to wash them. It'll make their colors bright. She held them up.

Be sure to clean the sink when you're through.

Dad already left for work. Would it be time for Neal to come home from school soon? They could go into the cookies then without asking. Neal had a big glass twice the regular size and would fill it up with milk. Dad used to tease him. Are you sure you have enough? And laugh.

But, even when Neal came, he wasn't going to stay inside. It was still light out. He would be going to meet his friends to play baseball before dinner. Today, when he came home he said they would be playing in the street in front of the house. Good! So, now she could watch. Neal would never take her to the schoolyard if they played there. The game was boring but sometimes she could help out by picking up a stray ball.

This time a lot of kids turned up. It was fun listening to them. They picked sides. Two big boys were signaling everyone to get out of the street when a car was coming. But soon, everyone had to leave. That meant it was time for dinner.

Since Dad wouldn't be there, Mom would probably give them the same old thing they'd had for lunch or something else cold. Maybe something different this time. Now you could smell fresh chopped onions and vinegar being mixed into some canned salmon. And Mom was letting them have those crisp salty shoestring potatoes from a can. A real treat! But even that favorite didn't work on her brother tonight. He seemed to be in a bad mood. He hadn't wanted to come in.

Can't we ever have hot food, something good for dinner when Dad isn't here?

Lily watched her mom. Her expression remained the same but you could feel a tightening. Mother took pride in not rais-

ing her voice. She told them that she never yelled in anger like
<u>her</u> mother.

Neal ate the dinner anyway. It was past six o'clock and
Captain Video already started. This show, the wall of the space
ship cabin had fallen down and there was a stage hand standing there, looking real surprised. She and Neal had burst out
laughing. The captain gave orders. Okay, Ranger, help me get
ready for lift-off, as they pulled the scenery back into place. At
six-thirty, there was no escaping the news. It was on every
channel. Another murder in Grant Park. Later tonight, *I Love
Lucy*, Mom's favorite, would be on. Neal didn't like sitting
with them and went to his room. Besides, he usually had
homework and then maybe would play with his crystal set.

When she followed him upstairs, he closed his door in her
face, leaving her standing next to the hall closet mirror. She
peered into the world behind her image. What would it be like
to walk through to those other rooms where everything would
be the same but opposite? Finally, she trudged over to her bed,
climbed up, just sat there, letting her legs dangle. Once Neal
had let her listen to the crystal set through earphones. It sounded very far away. It was hard to understand how this was a
radio.

Downstairs again, checking on the dining room, there was
nothing good on TV yet, only a game show. During Lucy, you
could hope for a snack, an ice cream Dixie cup and the wood-
en spoon it came with. On the inside, once you licked it clean,
the lid had a picture of a movie star. She had at least a dozen
in her collection. Next to Clark Gable, the best one was
William Powell. They both had mustaches. Veronica Lake and
her hair. She could never get enough ice cream if it was chocolate. And if it wasn't, Mom would open a can of chocolate
syrup.

At nine, after *I Love Lucy*, it was time for bed. The kitchen
clock which used to hang over the toaster had been moved a
long time ago. Now you could see it from the dining room
ticking away over the sink. She could already tell time and

Johnny, the boy next door, was six and still couldn't.

Her mother continued to sit in front of the TV, embroidering a linen napkin stretched in a hoop. Watching her sew for awhile, Lily then looked through the cigar box where skeins of thread in all the colors were lying next to each other. When she said her belly hurt, her mother told her to get some ginger ale. That will help you be less bloated. How could drinking all those little bubbles help?

Back up in her room, she would put on her nightgown. She was supposed to brush her teeth before going to bed. One time, Neal thought he put soap on her toothbrush. But it was her mother's. So he finally got caught. Now, she took off her clothes, carefully laying them out on a chair, including her panties, to wear again the next day. There was only one comfort left to her now. Maybe she would be kidnapped by an Arabian knight riding a camel. He would love her so much he had to have her with him and they would live in a tent.

It was lucky if she could fall asleep right away, even better to sleep through. Some nights, like this one, she woke up frightened. What was it that made her feel scared? But Dad must be home by now and the house was awfully quiet. Had she had a dream or was it the murder in the park? If she called out, he might get angry.

Finally, calling softly, then feeling braver with the sound of her own voice, she called again. Sometimes, he gave her a glass of water. Now, he turned on the elephant lamp. What's the matter?

What should she say? My stomach hurts.

How about if I give you some aspirin?

After it was chewed and washed down with a sip of water, he turned off the light. Go to sleep now.

When he had gone, she lay there in the dark listening to the wind getting louder, like it was coming from real far away. It was getting awfully noisy. Sneaking out of bed, she lifted a slat in the blinds. The glowing street lamp on its heavy concrete base seemed indifferent to the clumps of leaves and broken

217

branches swirling around it. Why should she feel so scared? She was *in* the house. Shivering from the cold and listening to the bottom slats rattle from the open window, she'd never fall asleep.

But she must have because now the sky was getting light. Hearing lonely sounds of fog horns on Lake Michigan and a train far away, what day was it? It couldn't be Sunday because Neal was in school yesterday. There was still a bad feeling in her stomach. Maybe it would be better if she ate some bread.

Mom and Dad were still asleep. She and Neal had to entertain themselves and keep quiet. Downstairs, he was already in the kitchen pouring milk into a bowl of cornflakes. He was getting ready to go to Danny's house where they were being allowed to set up Danny's new electric train permanently in the basement. Mom wouldn't let him keep his train out. Neal sounded disgusted. If it always had to be put away at the end of the day, it isn't even worth bringing it out. She remembered it taking forever just to lay the tracks. It might have taken a lot less time if he would let her help. But she couldn't touch any of his things—the Erector Set or Lincoln Logs. While she listened to him, she got the Rice Crispies out of the little metal cabinet along with the sugar bowl, never putting milk in dry cereal like Neal did.

Could she tell him about being scared last night? He would just make fun of her. Anyway, he was in a hurry, already zipping up his jacket. When he left, not knowing what else to do, she turned on the Saturday cartoons. It was Bugs Bunny because Road Runner was already over. Waiting for something good, she finally turned it off. There was talking upstairs now. What were they saying? It didn't sound nice. Sometimes Dad complained that Mom couldn't make dinner taste good. Like Grandma did.

While waiting for them to come down, she'd have a few cookies. It wasn't so windy now. Maybe she could ask Dad to take her to the park playground and zoo. He came down first.

Would you like some oatmeal? That she ate with milk and

salt. She didn't mind having breakfast again and it was okay with Dad. They were always telling her she was too skinny.

Daddy was too tired for the park today. They could go tomorrow on his day off. He had been promising 'soon' for a long time. Mom would be going shopping today and could pick up their special Sunday breakfast at the delicatessen. Then Dad wouldn't have to do it in the morning. Would she like to go shopping with Mommy? Neal would be at Danny's all day, Danny's parents driving him home in time for dinner.

Mom never ate oatmeal or cereal. Every day for breakfast, at exactly 9:30 she had coffee with milk and sugar, a roll, cream cheese, and lox or herring, moving from one thing to another without ever allowing an interruption. She'd read a newspaper while she ate. Today, with Dad and Lily waiting, Mom asked a question. After Thanksgiving, why couldn't they take a vacation to some place they hadn't been? Dad only wanted to go back to Wisconsin. Suddenly, Mom wouldn't say anything more. When the phone rang, she grabbed it. It must be Aunt Mary because Mom began complaining about Dad's not liking to go anywhere new. As soon as she hung up, the phone rang again and, answering it, Mother repeated what she had said during the other call. But who was it this time?

At first, they waited, expecting Mom to finish soon but then Dad said to Lily he had something for her. A customer had given it to him. He went to his coat in the closet by the front door. Returning, he handed her a small white cardboard box filled with cotton and, very carefully, helped her uncover three tiny glass dogs. Their shapes looked soft like clay but they were transparent except for their eyes, ears, and tongues. He smiled at her delight.

Her mother started to dial the phone again. Before she finished, Dad tried to get her to hang up and get ready to go, but you could feel Mom hanging back. Anyway, he had some drafting to do.

In the den, at his high work table, Lily stood across from where he sat on the stool and watched him making lines using the T-square and triangles. A strange triangular ruler had different numbers on each side. How did he keep the paper so clean? Even when he erased, there were never any smudges. They were plans for a house, he said, and he showed how different patterns meant brick or stone. Around the house, there were trees that looked like circles. He called it a bird's eye view. Arcs meant doors, double lines showed windows. He was surprised how she understood the drawing.

Finally tired of watching him, he let her look through a stack of old pictures. They were homes that seemed foreign, like cottages, not like houses up and down the street. So pretty, she tried to imagine the insides, like going through the mirror. Where were they? She never remembered to ask and he never said anything about them.

Hearing her mom go upstairs, he told her to go get dressed, too. It only took a minute. Then, standing at the bathroom door she watched Mom give herself a sponge bath at the basin, wiping the wash cloth under her arms, lifting each breast and washing there. Squeezing the water out of the cloth again, she washed her crotch, drying herself with the hand towel.

Her mother put on a girdle. It made Lily's belly hurt just to watch. Mom connected each hook and eye the whole length of it and, then, when it was holding her tight, she still had to work to zip it closed. Dangling from the girdle were garters in the front and back to hold up her nylons. It was beginning to get cooler, Mother said, so she could wear them. In the summer heat, she just put a flesh-colored cream on her legs that made it look like nylons. It all took so long.

Then, in the little bathroom downstairs, Mom would neaten her hair. Lily never saw her wash or brush it. The beauty shop did that. Mom would push a stray stiff brown curl into place, maybe using a hairpin or spraying it a bit. Then there was powder, rouge, and lipstick. She did look pretty.

It was getting late. Dad wondered if they hadn't better have lunch before they left.

I just finished breakfast. Lily can have a banana if she's

hungry.

It would be good to be away from the house, seeing people on the main street. They were supposed to be going to the deli but Mom would always look in a few stores on the way. And then maybe Lily would get another storybook doll or something from the dime store like a colorful 3-d plastic key chain puzzle.

Nowadays they had a new wheeled grocery carrier because there wasn't enough room in the buggy for the groceries and Lily. First stop was the post office on the corner, the big mail trucks pulled up along the side of the street the two of them had come from. As they walked past a narrow store with no windows, she peeked in the door that opened just as they went by. It was dark in there and it went way back. Men standing at a counter, loud music, and a familiar unpleasant stale odor. It made her think of Dad's liquor store and drunk men who were sometimes there.

Glad to get past it, the rest of the stores were bright and happier looking. Everything you could want. Mom stopped in a store with kitchen stuff.

Just looking around, she told the salesman. Comparing prices, she said to Lily after he left them, and Mom walked quickly in another direction. Always afraid of getting separated, Lily stuck close even if there was nothing interesting to look at. Strangely, this store had one locked glass cabinet high on a wall with several shelves of stuffed toy animals in it. They always stopped to look at them on the way out.

Mom had a shopping list written on scratch paper she made from tearing up letters that came in the mail. In the kitchen at home, the paper was kept along with short little yellow pencils in a flat drawer above the bread. Mom's writing was very tiny and curly not like the big waves of Daddy's writing but she couldn't read either of them, anyway. One day she had been pretending to write, imitating Neal. Dotting eyes and crossing tees, she'd asked him, does this spell anything? One time he said she wrote the word 'tea'. Very exciting, but, she wasn't able to do it again.

Looking in so many windows was taking a long time. When they actually went inside, they would go down every aisle. There didn't seem to be anything Mother would skip. The huge dime store in front of the movie theater was the best. Mom bought thread, a pattern, and some dishes of blue glass that matched the ones at home, then tried on some dresses, but didn't buy any. She would ask as she tried each one on, Do you like this? There were only certain clothing stores they could go in. Mom didn't like the ones with really fancy clothes, where you couldn't look at them yourself.

A department store on the way back was okay sometimes, maybe if there was a sale. That store was as big as three and it had a grand staircase leading to the basement. Near the bottom, the stairs split to the left and to the right. They always went to the right where there were more clothes and fabric, also a drinking fountain and bathrooms. There weren't any other bathrooms on the whole main street except in the restaurants and you had to order something.

Now, she felt tired, but Mom took her to the back of the store on the main floor. Shoes for the whole family.

You need some shoes.

The salesman was real nice, asked what she liked. Cowboy boots!

Out of the question. Too expensive.

She couldn't even try them on. The saddle shoes she picked were refused. I'd have to tie them for you. Loafers were okay, but they slipped off her heel.

Shoes with elastic gussets across the top. They stay in place.

When the elastic hurt, Mother got annoyed. Carefully fitting the shoes, the salesman then took her over to an x-ray machine that let them all look at the bones in her feet. This was supposed to prove that the shoes fit. She couldn't tell. None of them felt good.

More and more tired, could they go home soon?

The deli was crowded and Mom had to take a number. There was no place for her to sit. Food in the glass cases just made Lily more hungry. Rows of smoked fish, lox ready for slicing, herring, rolls, everything smelled so good. Her and her dad's favorite were onion rolls. Why couldn't she have one now? Mom just bought some along with a flat loaf of rye with caraway seeds. Still waiting for Mom, she watched chunks of halvah being hacked off for different customers. Mom hardly ever bought any of that. Her father, Grandpa Israel, brought some to them whenever he visited. A chunk of it would be in the brown bag filled with penny candy. He always handed this over before sitting down in the big blue satin brocade winged chair and going to sleep, cane hanging from the arm.

More and more hungry, she asked, Can I have a roll now? Not now, we'll stop at the Swedish bakery and I'll give you a quack-quack when we get there. Those were her favorite soft rolls that opened up like a duck's bill so you could butter them inside. But she and Neal never ate them with butter. She was shaky now, feeling weak.

At the Swedish bakery, they again had to wait for their number to be called. But at least there were padded benches where you could sit. Feeling worse and worse, she couldn't help beginning to cry. While Mom finished picking out a chocolate cake for Daddy and was waiting for the box to be tied, she finally handed over a roll.

Unable to stop crying, and licking the salty tears from her upper lip, she ate the roll with one hand and held onto the cart with the other, barely seeing where they were going. Mother said they would go to the drug store for a milkshake as soon as she was done in the grocery. The grocery! How could she wait any more?

Mom sat her on the wide window sill inside the front of the market. Wait here and take a rest. Milk, hot dogs, vanilla wafers for Neal, and more cottage cheese is all that is left to get.

Then, every time a woman with dark hair came to a check-out line, it seemed to be Mom. But it never was. Could Mom have left the store? Forgotten to pick her up? There had been a crash in the cookie aisle a little while ago. Maybe she dropped dead. Like Judge Goldberg.

Lily, about to begin crying again, saw Mom finally appear at a cash register and wave. Suddenly, everything was all right. While handing money to the clerk, the bag boy began walking to where Mom pointed. Hold the cake, Lily, while the nice man puts our groceries in the cart. Two big bags. Then Mom put the cake on top.

The small drug store/soda fountain was on the corner of their street, across from the post office. Feeling somewhat revived now, she walked to the apothecary counter at the back, like she usually did, to stare at the leeches. Why do doctors use them to suck blood? In other ways, the store was comforting with its oak cabinets and marble soda fountain. Sliding into a wooden booth, the soda jerk came right over to take their order. One cherry milkshake and two glasses. It only took a minute for the steel tumbler to arrive. Too thick to drink with a straw right away, she picked up the cellophane packet that held two sugar wafers, one chocolate, one plain. Mom always let her pick first.

Refreshed a little to make the trip home, they began the three-block walk. The first block always felt scary. Three-story apartment buildings and old elm trees made it dark and only people you didn't want to know lived there. The next block had thicker grass and more light. There were some friends on that block. Looking forward to their own block, almost all homes, even some empty lots where you could play with the older kids. They knew almost everyone and there always seemed to be more sunlight.

As they neared, they could see a fire engine and lots of people standing around. The Gimbel's house on the corner had flames shooting from an upstairs window, almost matching the glowing streaks of sunset behind it. She'd never seen a real fire before. Nothing exciting like that ever happened. Were people trapped in there burning up? There weren't any screams.

A neighbor spoke up, It was in a bedroom. An electrical wire in the wall. Just started by itself, he said. How could a fire start by itself? The neighbor was still talking. No one was in the bedroom so everyone was okay. After watching the firemen awhile, they walked home. Mother didn't say anything, but when Neal came home, she told him all about it. The Gimbel boys were there with their mother when it happened. As usual, he took it in without saying anything. Mom warmed the corned beef this time and they made their own sandwiches with the rye bread and mustard on the table. There was also a round white carton of cole slaw and new pickles wrapped in deli paper.

Now, Sid Caesar came on. Even Neal would watch. Staying up as late as they wanted on a Saturday, there wasn't anything else to do. Why did she want to stay up so late? She brought a throw pillow in from the living room and tried to watch TV while lying under the dining room table, but she was too tired. Her eyes kept going shut. No fire had ever happened in this house, but it could. You heard about them on the news. Her room was upstairs just like the Gimbels'. And her bed was next to the wall. What if she were asleep when her wall burst into flame? Mom and Dad might not even know it was happening. Tonight she would leave the elephant lamp on, even though she wasn't supposed to. And lie on the very edge of the bed.

-end-

Electricity

The butterfly counts not months but moments,
and has time enough.
- RABINDRANATH TAGORE

At the following visit, as soon as I entered Berry's room, she said, "I've been thinking. I don't like her having a dream about the fire."

I stood still for a moment trying to figure out what she was referring to.

As if to jog my memory, Berry said emphatically, "...the eyes of the dolls on the wall looking through the smoke..." Seeing that the bewildered look hadn't left my face she said more softly, "I liked that image at first—or am I ready for the loony bin?"

"Well, you usually *do* like what *you* write," I said and we both burst out laughing.

Berry had been rewriting in her head as she often did, only this time she had been rewriting my story. "I need to have you read the ending to me again," she concluded.

Something must not have been sitting well. However, when I finished re-reading it, Berry approved it as it stood. "But I've been thinking, if you're going to make these stories into an autobiography, you'll have to break them up and interweave them."

I groaned, imagining the amount of work it would take. As if reading my mind, Berry commiserated. "I know, it's a lot easier not to. Promise me you'll give my idea some serious consideration and I'll do the same for your notion of stringing them together chronologically."

More often, Berry was sending me away only a few minutes after I arrived. The amount of pain she was feeling depended on what time she had been given her pill, she told me. Once, when she didn't want to be bothered at all, even with greetings, she said sharply, "I can't work today. I'm too busy." She knew how to get me out of there quickly and smiling.

On my way to yet another part-time job, as I walked from my

car to the building, I gasped aloud as an electric pain ripped through my big toe. It felt as if I'd stepped on barbed wire and then tore my foot away. I stood riveted, peering down at my left sneaker. Balancing on my right foot, I lifted the left to examine the sole of the shoe. Nothing. What in the world could cause such pain?

It didn't happen again until a few days later. Once more, it made me gasp aloud. Only this time I was sitting in my car, getting ready to drive. My foot wasn't even touching anything except the shoe it was in. Over the next week it happened a few more times, each under different circumstances and with no indication of what was causing it.

The following week just after entering Berry's room, it happened again, my gasp startling Berry. I brushed it aside saying, "Just a pain I get in my foot sometimes."

Berry said "I have a new pain. It was so intense last night that I couldn't even reach up to hit the buzzer. I just lay here immobilized. It was like being electrocuted."

"Where was it?" I asked.

"In my feet and legs and stomach."

"Oh, that's terrible! Can the doctor change your medication?"

"I've been told they can't give me any more. How about giving me some sherry in one of those cups on the sink? Just half a cup."

This time I didn't hesitate. As I got the bottle out of the closet and poured some into the cup, I thought about Berry having been in the nursing home for almost a year-and-a-half, steadily getting weaker with increasing pain. A number of times Berry had said her feet felt like they were in boots that were being laced tighter and tighter.

I told her about the strange pain I'd been experiencing. "I'd describe it the same way you described yours. Electric! And tearing. And mine was just in one little spot—the end of my toe. A couple of times I've gasped so loudly out on the street that when other people were around, they jumped. I can't imagine what it would be like to feel something like that for hours throughout half of your body!"

I reminded Berry that in Byock's book, he discussed the need for hospice personnel to use medications that cut down on pain while keeping the patient lucid. "I'll see if I can get more information about drugs from him."

Regardless of Berry's terrible night, she was in the mood for talking. Her younger son would soon be moving to Virginia Beach. She was going to miss him and the children. Kathryn was keeping his kids for a few days during the actual move and then would drive them down to their new home.

I told Berry I had lived there for awhile almost thirty years before, working for the Edgar Cayce Foundation. "The area feels like a resort even though it's the biggest city in Virginia. It's because of all the waterways and the quality of light, I think." Then remembering an old friend of mine, I added, "I had a close friend there you would have gotten a kick out of. He was quite different from most people connected with the Foundation. He took particular pleasure in making the rest of us uncomfortable about our personas—you know, the false ways we sometimes present ourselves. I wrote a little vignette about him. Maybe I'll dig that out."

Berry was interested. "Bring it next time."

The night before I returned, I had a compelling dream:

I am looking down at a large yellow butterfly. Her hands keep reaching up to me. I let her touch me. When we are this close, I see she has the face of an old lady. I'm taken with her, continuing to feel her touch which tickles me. I wonder how old she is but don't ask, thinking it impolite. An old lady butterfly, after all, might be only a few days old in our time.

I want to give her a gift so I rummage through my jewelry drawer, searching for something colorful or glittery and at the same time meaningful. I find what looks to be an award pin, like the decoration a soldier or diplomat might receive. It has tiny rhinestone letters which spell out the word 'Learnéd.' The perfect gift!

When I saw Berry, I told her about my butterfly dream, realizing as I talked that I was looking down at her from the same angle I had been looking at old lady butterfly. Pleased with the dream, she smiled at me, invisible wings billowing softly.

The Seventh Story—Brute Sensitivity

Belief and Knowledge
Knowledge is something which you can use.
Belief is something which uses you.
- IDRIES SHAH

"I brought the story about Jim, my friend in Virginia Beach," I said, while displaying another delivery of hummus. Berry looked at the food instead of immediately reaching for it—as if debating about something.

Finally, she said, "Don't bring any more. Kathryn is providing her homemade hummus again, but I'll eat this as long as it's here. Would you crank up the bed? I can't seem to get comfortable today."

I crouched down at the foot, cranking and waiting for her to lift her hand in signal to stop. We fussed with the little black tubular pillow until Berry gave up trying to find the right place for it. She couldn't anymore. Although she enjoyed hearing about Jim and contributed comments to the writing, there was a sense that her discomforts were now beginning to overshadow even the last worldly pleasure of editing. We didn't work on it as long as the others.

Brute Sensitivity
Gazing through the glass partition into the press room at the

Foundation, I watched Richard, my boss at the new job, talking with a man I hadn't seen before. Who was that sinister-looking stranger? Even through the glass, his voice was getting louder as he announced needing to fix a scheduling conflict. He looked like a native from some exotic jungle. Curious, I went out to them.

When the wild man realized I was listening in on their conversation, he began making insinuating remarks to Richard.

And who is this, your handler?

Richard introduced us, This is Jim. He operates the presses. Unsmiling, Jim gave a piercing look and grunted acknowledgement. After their problem was resolved, Richard and I returned to our office.

Despite Jim's great gift for keeping the machinery running smoothly, his manner tested our endurance for discourteousness. Once again, I admired Richard's demeanor, his calm, and I couldn't help being somewhat intrigued by the dark-skinned man with long hair. For the moment, I returned to pasting up the book sales catalog with a photograph and description of each book. Where had the Foundation picked up such an untamed person?

In time, my laughing at Jim's baiting of our most proper co-workers must have endeared me to him. Maybe the only one who got his jokes. He amused me by challenging everyone's pretensions, including my own.

Subsequently, I was invited for dinner at his place where he was caretaker of a vacation home. I arrived with a contribution of homemade bread and a small bottle of wine. He graciously accepted the bread and handed the wine back to me.

I'm an alcoholic and haven't had a drink for years, he said gruffly, but you can drink it. Feeling it might be unpleasant for him, and not caring about it for myself, I put the bottle away in my bag.

In the entrance to his ground floor apartment was an immaculate three hundred gallon museum-quality aquarium teeming with a variety of brightly-colored fish. It must have been a lot of work keeping a tank that size healthy. I learned later that acquaintances had given it to him. They knew it would be cared for and used to its full potential.

Everything in Jim's apartment was tended to and had been positioned with care, including the parallel cigarette butts in the moderne turquoise ashtray. There was a distinct feeling that many of the furnishings were hand-me-down. The tropical theme ran throughout. Would I have guessed he'd have bamboo furniture with colorful plant patterns on the cushions, decorative fishing nets and sea shells on the walls? Most of us living year around in the Virginia Beach community and working at the Foundation didn't have a lot of money. First garbage day after the tourist season provided us all with a hoard of exotic furnishings.

What made Jim look so sinister? Dark skin with shiny long black curly hair, pulled back severely in a pony tail long before (or after) this was an acceptable style. You could see he had a gentle side—tied his hair with a ribbon! Every day it was a different electric color, matching his socks and t-shirt. Artistic, kind of raw—like a painting on black velvet. His harshness was a bluff, just a litmus test for friendship....

"Intelligence," Berry broke in. I wrote it in and reread the sentence.

....His harshness was a bluff, just a litmus test for friendship, or was it intelligence?

Rarely smiling at work, he would pointedly refer to the foibles or internal contradictions of any of us who talked with him. Instructive as it was, the overall effect was often intimidating, making him somewhat unpopular. He had fans, though, who appreciated his brutal perception, even finding it refreshing amidst the prevailing politeness that surreptitiously kept everyone at a distance from each other.

Conveying the notion that he preferred things to people, he would, nevertheless, hold free classes teaching us how to do basic maintenance on our cars or how to change a tire. Sometimes he earned his living repairing automobiles. He'd already worked on my car when a minor spark plug problem surfaced. Watching him test the wires, it was a surprise to see his hands move so deftly, like a surgeon. When he disconnected a wire, I expected to see blood flow. Auto maintenance never before seemed to be an art, but watching Jim work on cars was like watching a potter or a painter, awakening a sense of the sacred.

He took pleasure in some of my mechanical troubles. I'd just had my sewing machine repaired for it's slipping clutch when my car was also diagnosed with a clutch affliction.

Looks like you need to get a grip, he mocked. Haven't you noticed how our machines reflect our internal state of being?

As he grew into a dependable friend, Jim and I would share an occasional meal, spend time together at work, and show each other discoveries in books we read.

After having lived in Virginia Beach for about fifteen months, I received a letter from Mr. Bennett, the man I had studied with in England, asking if I'd join with other students of his in founding an intentional community in West Virginia. It was to be based on the principles we learned when we studied with him and would include establishing a school. I agreed to move there.

Just a couple of months before leaving, I received a mysterious phone call from a local friend who had also studied with Bennett. What was he calling about? He didn't want to tell me over the phone. Having to be at work that day and the next, I couldn't meet with him when he wanted. What is it? Reluctantly, he told me that Mr. Bennett had died suddenly.

I thought back to the day at his school when one of the students asked Bennett if he intended, after five years of having the school at Sherborne, to begin another community like the one he'd had for fifty years in Kent. Bennett laughed, shaking his head, blue eyes twinkling. "I hope I never have to live in a community like that again," he said. Damned if he hadn't found a way out.

I was shocked by his death, however, because he hadn't been sick. I learned that only a few hours before lying down to take his last nap, he'd been wheelbarrowing through the garden. I could picture him in his houndstooth jacket with the brown leather patches on the elbows, tall, imposing, white haired, eyes set on finishing whatever task he had going. Grateful to him for having infused new energy into my life during our studies back then, now, I went to my room to cry, wondering if the community in West Virginia would still happen. Soon after, I learned that his students were going ahead with plans for Claymont.

At Jim's house a couple of days after Bennett's death, I distractedly asked him for a piece of paper.

There's this image that's been trying to make itself known to me, I muttered, holding back a surprising urge to cry. It just came again—a little more clearly this time.

Jim sat quietly, watching me draw. What the hell was this? It looked like a sunny side up egg, yolk and white, except the whole thing was teardrop shaped. Mr. Bennett, dead. Feel sad. He's just fine, happy, he says. I'm glad to have known him.

All this while, I'd said nothing aloud to Jim who was thoughtfully watching as I drew. Then, grabbing a book from the bookcase, he riffled through the pages. What was he looking for? The book was a volume of Besant and Leadbeater's *Thought Forms*. Not yet having said anything about what was going on in my mind, I was amazed when he showed me some pictures and text. Fig. 34 was labeled 'At A Funeral'. It consisted of two pictures showing what the authors purported to be thought forms over two mourners contemplating death. (illustrations after p.71, words p.52) One was muddy colored and described as "vague, depressed, selfish". The other, a teardrop shaped egg, as having "most beautiful sentiments."

The book stated, "This knowledge (of theosophy) takes away all fear of death, and makes life easier to live because we understand its object and its end, and we realize that death is a perfectly natural incident in its course, a necessary step in our evolution. There is no gloomy impenetrable abyss beyond the grave, but instead of that a world of life and light which may be known to us as clearly and fully and accurately as this physical world in which we live now."

How could something I experienced so subjectively be illustrated and discussed in this book as if it were objective? And how had Jim gone right to it among all the books he had on his shelves? I was befuddled, elated, and comforted.

-first ending-

Berry had interrupted me only once during that reading so we assumed the story was finished. However, her interest in Jim got us talking more about him. She asked, "Do you still know him?"

That's when I revealed one more incident relating to Jim and I wrote it up for the next visit.

During a period of ten years I had left Virginia Beach as planned, lived at the intentional community for three-and-a-half, returned to Chicago for another three, earning a social work degree and getting married. Bruce and I moved to West Virginia not far from the community, about three hundred miles north of Jim who had remained in Virginia Beach. He and I still corresponded regularly, though infrequently.

In his latest letters he had enclosed striking photographs of lotus blossoms and water lilies he was growing in the ponds of the new meditation garden at the Foundation. He'd moved in with a group of people who had land which allowed him to garden freely. I was glad he had found some kindred spirits who valued him.

Bruce and I had moved at the end of summer and it was already December. Knowing I still owed Jim a letter and having repeatedly put off writing, I was feeling sorry to have been so preoccupied. Finally having found a house to rent, my husband and I reclaimed our abundant belongings stored in a friend's basement and put the house in order. One night, having already turned out the bedroom lights, I tossed and turned in the moonlight streaming through the window until, I can't say how, Jim seemed to be urging me out of bed. I grudgingly dragged myself to the dining room to write him the long over-due letter which I mailed first thing in the morning.

Not hearing back immediately didn't concern me, but I began thinking of him often, with an odd feeling of anxiety. In front of my mailbox a month after I'd written to him, I pulled out a letter with a return address showing his last name and Marion, Ohio. Immediately, my heart sank. That's where Jim's family lived. Maybe he's visiting home, I tried telling myself. It was from his father, saying that my letter to Jim had been for-warded to him. 'It is very sad that it is necessary that I have to report to you of son Jim's death on Sept 18th...' Jim had a hemorrhage from coughing—tuberculosis. His friends found him in the garden, too late. Surely suspecting he was fatally ill, he would have avoided going to a hospital, preferring to die in more sympathetic surroundings.

-end-

Reading to Berry

A rock pile ceases to be a rock pile
the moment a single man contemplates it,
bearing within him the image of a cathedral.
- ANTOINE DE SAINT-EXUPERY, FRENCH AUTHOR, AVIATOR

Berry and I didn't talk any more about Jim. There was a sense we were done working on stories. Her energy had become too errat-ic, yet she still had occasional projects.

"I'd like to dictate a letter to my granddaughter." In it, she did

235

not directly answer a question Sybil apparently posed regarding the wisdom of living at home or at school. "Pray for enlightenment," Berry counseled, "You must know that genius has desperate antisocial requirements. I pray that such a fate will not befall you."

I could only guess. Did Sybil think living at home was distracting her from fulfilling her genius? If Berry had wanted to talk about it she would have. She treated her family's business with respect.

Before I left that day, Berry asked, "Do you have any books by Jung that discuss the shadow?"

"I have a couple but the easier one to understand would be *Man And His Symbols*. That was written for the lay reader by Jung and three of his students. I can't understand his professional writings, though you probably would."

At our next meeting, I read excerpts about the shadow, Berry having me read them over again immediately.

> This is the concept of the "shadow," which plays such a vital role in analytical psychology. Dr. Jung has pointed out that the shadow cast by the conscious mind of the individual contains the hidden, repressed, and unfavorable (or nefarious) aspects of the personality. But this darkness is not just the simple converse of the conscious ego. Just as the ego contains unfavorable and destructive attitudes, so the shadow has good qualities—normal instincts and creative impulses....

Then, from a caption next to a photo of Jewish prisoners after the Warsaw uprising:

> Repressed unconscious contents can erupt destructively in the form of negative emotions—as in World War II.

In a different section was another paragraph Berry asked to hear twice:

> Modern man does not understand how much his "rationalism" (which has destroyed his capacity to respond to numinous symbols and ideas) has put him at the mercy of the psychic "underworld." He

has freed himself from "superstition" (or so he believes), but in the process he has lost his spiritual values to a positively dangerous degree. His moral and spiritual tradition has disintegrated, and he is now paying the price for this break-up in world-wide disorientation and dissociation.

"Would you photocopy those pages so I can give them to my grandson?" Berry asked.

Occasionally Berry still mentioned writing a story about a nursing home since the first story had lived a life of its own and gone astray. She initiated a new tale one day, but after two pages, left it, never wanting to work on it again. As her energy was depleted so quickly, I more often read to her.

I also began a quiet campaign to learn something about her medications, writing down the names. I emailed Dr. Byock who promptly answered, recommending a brand new book that discussed the latest in pain technology.

Pain Control

Take the first step in faith.
You don't have to see the whole staircase, just take the first step.
- DR. MARTIN LUTHER KING JR.

Power Over Pain: How To Get The Pain Control You Need by Eric M. Chevlen M.D. and Wesley J. Smith, followed conventional medical protocol, something we could not do on our own. I suggested giving it to Berry's doctor. "No," she admonished. "He'll just keep it and not actually use it. Then we won't be able to get to it at all."

When I phoned Mary Jane, our hospice nurse friend who had

introduced us, and told her what Berry was being given, she said, "Those aren't the best medications. We should be able to control the pain and keep her alert. You mean that hospice isn't involved after all this time?" she asked.

"I didn't know hospice could be involved with someone in a nursing home. Why would we want them to be?" I asked.

"Because her doctor, who is quite old, may tend to use the same meds he's always used whereas hospice makes an effort to keep up with new practices. Why don't you call Kathryn and Berry's doctor and see if he'll refer her to hospice?"

Kathryn was willing yet dubious. "Isn't Mom just wanting to be drugged-up like she was with alcohol all those years?" It was a fair question.

Phone calls to the doctor's office were fruitless, the doctor never available and never returning my calls. Finally, he left a message for me with his staff saying Berry wasn't ready for hospice, that if they used it now, there wouldn't be any funding left for when she *really* needed it.

How could she need it more than now? Couldn't he see that she was unable to function any more? But from his distant view she hadn't been functioning for a year-and-a-half. He didn't spend the kind of time with her that would make the differences apparent.

After a couple more weeks of phoning, suddenly I found myself speaking with the doctor. As if just waiting to be asked, he said, "Of course I can put her in hospice. No problem."

Berry wanted to hear some of the writing in books I had called inspiring. In Ken Carey's *The Third Millennium*. he described being in bed with a fever, "feeling more elated than ill." He said that if the voice he heard hadn't been so reasoning, he might not have made it through the experience. The feeling was one of coming into focus after a lifetime of double vision or of finding some eternal part of himself he had forgotten. Since he could barely read his own handwriting when he tried to write what was being said, he pulled out an old manual portable typewriter his brother-in-law had found on a curbside years before.

I found myself experiencing a consciousness radically different from anything I had ever before encountered. And it was too close for comfort. I felt as if something enormous were looking through my eyes, seeing the same room I saw every day but interpreting it so differently—mathematically, it seemed—that I hardly recognized even the most familiar of my daily objects. The thoughts, the ideas, the scope of the images—I was not used to thinking in such terms.

Since the Careys had no electricity and a snow storm had bent the trees across the road, they were essentially cut off from the outside world for the eleven days it took him to receive this strange transmission. Previously, he had not known how to type, but that didn't stop him from producing 350 pages of a spiritual vision—"and my life had forever and irreversibly changed," he stated.

Berry, fascinated with Carey's experience of a higher consciousness dictating to him a manual for awakening and making an evolutionary leap, was, nevertheless, unable to concentrate for more than a few pages at a time.

The doctor increased her morphine which allowed her to sleep. When we spoke, however, Berry explained to me that it didn't really stop the pain.

"It just lets me retreat into my inner world. Talking with you brings me out of it and then I'm aware of the pain again. Only if I've received the pill about half an hour before you come am I actually without pain for a short time."

"Let's talk with the doctor and see if he can do something better."

Berry looked at me with disgust. "No! Let me drift. Some days I just don't want to talk. Leave me alone!"

She was unyielding. There was nothing to do but go away.

Still, she had times where she enjoyed a short chat and being read to. At those moments, she was alert and her usual witty self. It just didn't last very long. I never saw her eat, and, in passing, one day Kathryn said to me with frustration, "I don't know why she refuses to eat." Berry was still in charge of herself.

For a couple of weeks, she allowed me to read from another book, *Other Ways of Knowing: Recharting Our Future With Ageless Wisdom* by John Broomfield, the past president of the California Institute of Integral Studies. She enjoyed his remarkable perceptions, nodding and smiling after the most moving passages.

Broomfield's Book

If knower and known were made of different stuffs,
there could be no direct relationship between the two.
- J.G. BENNETT, THE DRAMATIC UNIVERSE

"Where did you find this book?" Berry wanted to know.

"I met the author at Omega. I was taking a five-day music workshop and we were invited to take an evening at another workshop we might be interested in for the future. John Broomfield was the facilitator. He seemed to be able to describe a view of life that was difficult to put into words. When I learned he'd written a book, I searched for it. So dense, it's not easy reading."

That was the right thing to say. Berry wanted to hear it. I just read excerpts knowing her energy couldn't last very long.

The Present Shapes the Past
History is not a set of facts fixed in the past, simply awaiting proper selection and ordering. History is the present perception of past events. There is no history apart from the "historian." The observer and the observed past are inextricably entwined.

The Limits of History
....In fact, linear time and sequential cause and effect are merely two of the patterns we have constructed in order to make sense of reality. Like all such explanatory patterns they are simplifications of the

universe, which, in its inconceivable vastness and complexity, is always threatening to overwhelm the limited capacity of the human organism to comprehend.

The Word

....Our history provides for modern Western civilization a view of reality alien to those who recognized other living creatures—and goddesses, gods, and spirits—as occupying places of prominence in their world. It is the consciousness of these ancestors that informed human experience down the long millennia, and our narrowly focused man-history is a barrier to our empathy with that experience.

My former Michigan colleague, Kathryn Reid, a Sioux, recounts how shocked she was in her first weeks in elementary school to discover that her white teacher was innocent of the fact that trees have lessons to teach us. Interspecies communication, at the heart of Native American life and of many other peoples, does not loom large in standard American or European school curricula or in our history books. For our culture it is not real.

Berry conversed for a short time one day, suddenly asking me what I was currently working on.

"I'm thinking of a new class. I'll call it, *Afraid of Art? Make Something Useless.*" That was the last hearty laugh we shared.

The next time I came, there was a hearse parked in front of the nursing home. Was it for Berry?

When I entered her room, she showed me she was still alive, quickly making it clear she did not want to be disturbed. I continued to call on her, sometimes sitting a short while if she were oblivious of my presence. If conscious, she would thank me for coming and wave me away, often angrily. "You people just interrupt me in the comfort of my inner world," she complained. I felt like I failed her in not finding a way to rid her of the pain.

Yet she told me in no uncertain terms, "I welcome the drug haze and maybe my soul even benefits from my physical suffering—paying a debt for my transgressions."

On a following visit, she greeted me saying, "I was in pain the whole night. I just had the morning pain pill so sit quietly while it takes effect and then we can talk."

I happened to glance down, noticing Berry's red pain pill contrasting sharply against the black and white speckled floor . When an aide came in asking Berry how she was, I pointed to it, saying, "Berry tells me she was in pain the whole night." Slowly comprehending, the woman picked it up, quietly telling me she would bring it to a nurse.

At home, I phoned Mary Jane and asked her what I should do. "Call hospice and tell them what happened. Ask them if they think they could help." Hospice needed to speak with Kathryn. I was not family.

Late the next afternoon, Kathryn phoned me, distraught. "Last night I had Mom brought to the emergency room. She was furious with me. It hurt her so much to be moved. I knew it was useless but I had to do something. It's clear she's dying." Kathryn had been with her mom all day and was exhausted. She asked, "Could you come later and sit with her?"

I arrived at 8:40 p.m. to find Kathryn weeping, talking on the phone with the doctor. Berry's body lay like an uninhabited sea shell on the shore. When Kathryn hung up, she said, "Mom died at 7:50." She stood and we hugged each other, crying. "May I use your arrival as an excuse to go home now? Would you wait for the funeral attendants to come?"

"Of course," I said and Kathryn, still distraught, hurriedly swept through the room, gathering only a few items.

Classical music that Berry loved still blared from the boom box. Kathryn's brief case, laptop, cell phone, and papers were spread on the chairs and window sill. I turned off the stereo and sat with Berry, unable to sense her presence. I wished I could have been with her. I tried to get the jangling energy in the room settled but didn't succeed. No matter, the men from the funeral home, dressed in their dark suits, soon arrived.

While they prepared to take Berry's corpse, I went to the nurses' office. "Would you lock up Kathryn's belongings?" I asked.

The nurse said, "I'd prefer your taking them with you. They'll be safer," she explained.

I returned to Berry's room just as the men were wheeling the gurney out. Standing in the hall, watching, I said, "Goodnight." Then I walked back in and slowly gathered Kathryn's things, still trying to create a sense of quiet by putting them in order.

Early the next morning, I phoned Kathryn to let her know where her possessions were. Then I called Mary Jane and Lynn, who had been alternating visiting days with me until Berry had sent her away. They both were relieved to hear that Berry's ordeal was finally over.

Midday, Kathryn and another family friend came by, transferring everything from my trunk to Kathryn's car. The three of us strolled around the garden languidly taking in the June flowers, talking about Berry, and the possibility of having lunch together some time. The serenity of the moment made me remember once when Berry said she hoped I could become friends with her daughter, knowing how difficult it was for her to take time for herself.

Berry's Memorial

Why do writers write? Because it isn't there.
- THOMAS BERGER

Kathryn asked me to speak at Berry's memorial service. It would take place over a month later, giving family and friends time to arrange travelling from afar. I was fearful of speaking in public, but I knew this was something I had to do. I'd been lucky to have spent so much time talking with Berry about her favorite subject.

When I bumped into Georgia, the friend who had lived with Berry many years ago, she asked me about Berry's last days.

"When she was close to dying, she couldn't tolerate anyone,

including me. I know she could be so abrupt and grating, but I seem to have received her best. With me, she was patient and encourag..."

"Berry seemed to have fallen in love with you," Georgia exclaimed with a hint of sharpness. We laughed. It was true and it was mutual. Once home again, I picked up *The Mystic Adventures of Roxie Stoner* and gazed at Berry's picture, reminded again of her challenging stare. (As I write this I can hear her say, Change the word 'challenging'. I answer, 'Wall-eyed comes to mind' and makes me laugh but it peeves her. The challenge is in the mouth; in the eyes, there's more of a sadness. Maybe you're sorry you have to make demands. And then, there's an impishness in the lines at the outer corners of those intense eyes, as if you're tempted to laugh at us for letting you intimidate us.)

The memorial was held in a restaurant banquet hall. At the far end of the room facing a podium were rows of chairs with a center aisle, arranged to feel like a chapel. Close to the door, along the wall, tables displayed books, articles, and pictures of Berry. Before seating ourselves, the chairless end of the room teemed with people, everyone introducing themselves to each other and sharing stories about Berry punctuated with laughter.

Almost a dozen speakers offered tales of friendship, writing, and challenges posed by their relationships with her. One colleague recalled the moment he first met Berry. She showed up at her new job in academia wearing the gum boots she wore for her work with the cows earlier that day. I recalled her telling me about being snubbed for her lack of credentials. This must have been her way to rub it in.

Kathryn's stalwart husband said, "As hard a time as she gave me, I know if she had *really* wanted to chase me away, she was capable of doing so." Berry had told me many times she thought him to be a genius, yet that never stopped her from always being hard on him, rubbing salt in whatever wounds she could produce or discover.

A Catholic priest, Father D., who performed opening and closing prayers also spoke of Berry's paradoxical character, her suffering no fools and loving God.

I let the mourners know that Berry's remarkable intellect had been active until the end.

"The story Berry meant to have been about a nursing home," I told them, "had quickly been usurped by a pushy self-centered character, who steered the action around him in an unplanned direction. Until then, I had only heard anecdotes from writers about characters who determined the story they were in, regardless of the author's intentions. After Berry finished that story, she still wanted to write about a nursing home because, as she put it, 'The topic provides so much humorous material.'

"About three weeks before she died she uncharacteristically, for that time, greeted me excitedly.

"'I've got the title for my story!' she exclaimed.

"'What?' I asked, absurdly thinking she'd begin writing again.

"'I'll call it *The Last Resort.*'"

For the half year following Berry's death, I taught a few more adult education classes and substituted in the public schools, but my heart wasn't in any of it. Each time there was an opportunity to sign up for more, I opted out. Then, I gave up volunteering for the practitioners' network and did nothing to move the Healing Arts Council to action. Instead, against all reason and responsibility, the idea of writing a book dominated my thoughts.

Just before the New Year, I heard the thought that surely I could devote January through March only to writing.

You could finish the first draft in that amount of time.

What about earning a living? I muttered to myself.

Well, you're not earning one anyway, just spending your small retirement fund. Do you want to be eking along in your dotage, still needing to work yet never having even tried to write a book?

So I began, never thinking about self-discipline unless a friend asked. Maybe writing came more naturally than I realized. As an artist, I had never been that devoted. I had been equally focused when I'd written the newsletter—and that demanded, what in some people creates greater resistance, a deadline. I'd prepare for each day just as when I'd been employed, the difference being that writing made me happy.

I spent most of the day writing, taking breaks by gardening or talking with friends on the phone, meditating, varying activity according to what felt needed—a natural rhythm. My digestion calmed down. I couldn't remember ever having been so centered.

At the end of March, the first draft was finished as planned— well over 500 pages. After reading it straight through for the first time, I felt glued to the sofa, disappointingly dazed. When finally able to move, I phoned Tara. "Why doesn't it work?" I asked. She listened patiently to my rambling. "I'd done it the way I'd told Berry I was going to—arranging the stories chronologically, moving from the childhood that established my pessimism through the events that challenged it. It contained everything I've felt touched by, including Berry, plus a lot more mystery than what I'd told her. But, in the end, it reads like a list, not literature."

War In Iraq

I like to believe that people in the long run
are going to do more to promote peace than our governments.
Indeed, I think that people want peace so much
that one of these days governments had better get out of the way
and let them have it.
- DWIGHT DAVID EISENHOWER (1890 - 1969)

Tara softly encouraged me to give the draft more consideration. "We'll talk again," she said.

After I hung up, I heard a thought in my head saying, You had chosen pessimism.

What do you mean? I asked, suddenly indignant over something I knew to be true.

No experience was good enough, that is, convincing enough for you to truly let it into your life. Do you believe you were touching another reality or not?

Of course, I believe it! I felt it. I cherished each event, collected them throughout my life.

Yet never acting on them—at least not until you finally realized that you needed to cultivate optimism. It no longer came naturally. Remember what I said? Fear and belief cannot co-exist. Trust the experience.

Pessimism is based on facts, I countered, as if still needing to be right.

Only on chosen ones, like poor science you so eloquently spoke to me about, ignoring what doesn't fit the paradigm. Remind me, what does pessimism get you? she asked gently.

Despair. That's what it got me. Just the opposite of those special events which always made me feel embraced by Love, connected to something greater, often offering insight and compassion beyond my own perception.

Turning my thoughts to the purpose of the book I was trying to write, I realized Berry had been correct about the structure. The stories needed to be woven together differently—with a better-defined objective. What about in the context of our friendship?

Was that the sound of her chuckling?

At the time I was finishing the first draft, the U.S. was considering war in Iraq. There seemed a shift in consciousness trying to break through. Whether people supported the war or not, there was a growing expression of aspiring to peace—prayer for intervention by spiritual powers, wishing for the health of all people, eschewing blame, seeking solutions.

When the U.S. entered Iraq, someone asked if I would alert our local email list of a silent vigil being held nearby. They would be praying for success in disarming Iraq of weapons of mass destruction; the safety and welfare of U.S. military; the welfare of their families; the well-being of the people of Iraq; and the peace and security of the world. A few people emailed me thanks for letting them know of the vigil. However, when I opened a certain email, its ferocity, like a strong headwind, blew me against the back of my chair.

What's wrong with you people? How about praying and giving thanks for a president that knows the Lord Jesus Christ as his Savior and isn't afraid to say so? This is just another Bush-bashing posing as a peace march.

The uninvited hostility almost shoved me into a canyon of despair when suddenly I heard Berry laughing. Remember what Carl Sandburg wrote? she asked. 'Sometime they'll give a war and nobody will come.' I decided, instead, to join her amusement.

The Second Draft

We are cups, constantly and quietly being filled.
The trick is, knowing how to tip ourselves over and
let the beautiful stuff out.
- RAY BRADBURY

Home repairs, spring gardening, and a trip to Chicago necessitated by Bruce's job intervened with writing. I fretted.

You know, I'd always recommended taking a break. It was hard to get you to take one back then and it's hard now, Berry reminded me. I stopped worrying.

After a couple of months of the manuscript simmering on the back burner, however, I began waking up in the middle of the night with ideas about rearranging the material. Sometimes I would awaken writing and rewriting sentences in my head, suspiciously in the manner Berry used to describe.

A technique I've been teaching you, the Berry-thought said. Sign up for a writing class. It's free to you instructors.

I joined a class for people who had manuscripts. We listened to each other read from our work and were guided by Kathleen, the instructor, on how to give feedback in a helpful way.

"You have no dialogue," one of the students pointed out. I'd never written dialogue. The closest I'd ever come was in quoting people I had interviewed for the newsletter. For the next class, I wrote pages of dialogue, desperately in need of interruption. Listening to myself read made it apparent.

My classmates asked questions.

"Where is this taking place?"

"What do the characters look like?"

"How old are they?"

"What gestures do they make?"

They laughed where it was funny or praised the painting of a scene with a good phrase. Still so much more to learn! I newly appreciated Berry's patience. Why, she'd barely broken ground in getting me to write literature.

It was fun and you're a hard worker, the Berry-thought said, again, encouragingly.

Kathleen suggested, "Read the kind of books you want to write."

I'd never realized that almost the only kind of book I read aside from those on alternative health care were memoirs or novels that sounded like them—*The Distant Land Of My Father, The Notebook, The Secret Life of Bees, White Oleander.*

I was always wondering how people lived their lives. What were their strengths? What were the conditions they lived under? What had each one been required to learn in order to accomplish what they did? What unplanned help came to them? As I furiously embarked on rearranging the book material, Rob Brezsny's August horoscope arrived by email:

Gemini. Do you think you'd enjoy being able to focus all your ambitions in one overarching dream? Can you imagine what it might be like not to feel your desires split in five different directions? While your predilection for versatility and vacillation isn't necessarily a bad thing, Gemini, it might be interesting at some point in your life to explore the ferocious pleasures of single-mindedness. It so happens that now is a perfect moment to launch such an exploration. Mars, the planet that rules willpower and determination, is currently expressing tremendous force in your astrological House of Total Commitment. There has rarely been a better time for you to stabilize your purpose and steel your resolve.

In the fall, instead of signing up for Kathleen's next class, I asked her for a few private sessions to read sections to her that I identified as troublesome. She invited me to her house, suggesting we work at the dining room table. As we passed through the living room I noticed several foxes—a folk sculpture and needlepoint pillows. In the dining room were dozens more, even some toy ones she said were from her childhood. I hadn't thought of her as a totem respecting person.

"Before we get started, why don't you pick a medicine card?" she asked in a playful voice, while holding a bowl in front of me. I dipped my hand into the cards and poked around, pulling one out. Turning it over, I read, "Wolf." The illustration showed a howling wolf's head with the moon behind it and five ornaments hanging below the shield that was its circular frame. The ornament furthest to the left was a brown striped feather! I read the rest of the inscription. *Find new paths & options. Break through. Be a role model. Share your inner knowing.*

In answer to my questions about writing, Kathleen pointed me in new directions. More ideas about the manuscript perked into consciousness.

Every time I felt stuck, I'd phone Tara who would patiently wade with me through the latest dilemma, sometimes suggesting a solution or a new angle, sometimes a particular book about writing. Occasionally, she would read something to me for inspiration.

By the end of December, I had refined the second draft.

Brezsny was right! I'd never experienced such single-mindedness in my whole life. In sixty-one years, it had never even been an option.

While still working on that draft, I thought, Had it been a waste of time writing so many pages that were cut?

That's not what I said! Berry sounded annoyed.

Well, I just don't describe things the same way you do. We're still having fun with words, aren't we? But I couldn't hide sounding vexed. She'd taken me by surprise even if it was in my own head.

Yes, we are, she said hesitantly. Then she muttered, Admitting it, though, detracts from the power of scolding. Then she warned me, Don't drift into using quotation marks for any more discussions. You've used them for hundreds of pages.

I promise, I said too quickly and just as quickly asked myself how I was going to show the difference between an outer conversation and an inner thought. Before Berry could say more, I rationalized meekly, I hadn't been using them in the first person present tense flashbacks or in the stories we wrote together or in your comments since you died.

That's a start, she agreed. Then she informed me, We're pretty much eliminating the first person present tense flashbacks, anyway. They're too complicated. Maybe we'll save a few dreams. No reader wants to work that hard to figure out what's going on.

In the second version of *The Transparent Feather*, I thought I'd achieved the single purpose of supporting the theme of the creative relationship between Berry and me. In fact, our alliance was still going on. Hadn't I once wondered if I'd even enjoy writing without her?

In the spring, Kathleen started a read-and-critique group. I had readily agreed to join, yet I wondered if it was the best use of time. When Tara and I arrived at Kathleen's house, on the street behind my parked car was a damaged yellow butterfly. I maneuvered it onto my palm and brought it into the meeting to show everyone. It tickled me, feeling exactly as the old lady butterfly had in my dream. Could I take its presence as a sign of being in the right place? I thanked it and released it into the bushes.

More Feedback

The most powerful thing you can do
(and it is very powerful)
to change the world is to change your own beliefs
about the nature of life, people, and reality,
and begin to act accordingly.
- SHAKTI GAWAIN

I struggled with the deficit of quotation marks and finally pulled Berry's book, *The Mystic Adventures of Roxie Stoner*, off the shelf to see how she did it.

Damn! She has quotation marks. What was she talking about?

Only in the first eight chapters, chided Berry. Remember, *Roxie* was originally a series of short stories. I changed my style. Looks like my editor missed making them consistent. I think quotes are an unnecessary complication. It's a good exercise for you to make do without them. Keep it up.

I huffed in exasperation.

Reflecting my increasing dedication to optimism, I read the comics daily. Their descriptions of human foibles and politics were so much more perceptive than journalism. News gave no support to admirable work that people were doing against all odds. Popular media behaved as if its job was to purposely stir up anger and indignation. Spreading ill will should be a crime, I thought. Groups like the Interfaith Encounter Association who regularly sponsored mixed Christian, Jewish, Islamic, and Druze gatherings in Israel never made the news.

I'm glad to see you using your internal compass, Berry noted, in your case, your emotions. When you're being fed attitudes that make you angry or overwhelmed, it's a sure sign it's time to change your diet.

She's become a health maven!

Thinking back to a time when I thought all optimistic people were naive, Berry corrected me. You only attended to the Pollyannas who refused to see what was wrong. Now you recognize true optimists—people who recognize something that isn't right and use their imaginations to make life better in whatever way they can.

Had I meant it when I used to tease the social worker at an earlier job ten years ago, calling her *pathologically optimistic*? I had at first. Then it became clear she really made a difference. She always developed a loving rapport with the people we advocated for, listening to them and finding a way to support their goals.

I had been drawn to Berry, hoping that her intelligence, wisdom, and closeness to death would help me live more fully. At that time, I still had no sense of expressing a unique purpose I felt inside.

A thought came as if she were speaking, You're such an intelligent person. Really, all you needed from me was the experience of someone appreciating your gifts.

J.G. Bennett

Frisbeetarianism is the belief that when you die,
your soul goes up on the roof and gets stuck.
- George Carlin

As if needing to talk with Berry about what was going on I

explained to her in my head, Thirty years ago, my search had led to my studying with J.G. Bennett in England. As had happened in the past, certain interactions with him are now urgently returning to my awareness unbidden.

His career had brought him to the near and far East where he had met with several respected spiritual teachers. Eastern religions, he explained, have a significantly more detailed understanding of the holy architecture of the body and how to access it to enhance spiritual life.

You know what, Berry? I'm going to use quotes. It just feels clearer to me to know immediately that a person is talking aloud.

As long as your purpose is clear to you, Berry answered. You never *have* to do what I suggest.

She was grinning.

"Eastern religions," he explained, "have a significantly more detailed understanding of the holy architecture of the body and how to access it to enhance spiritual life."

That's better. See?

The Berry thought acknowledged my point, not necessarily agreeing with it.

He shared with his students meditative exercises he thought would be especially useful for us, living now in Western culture.

"One of the structures—the five sacred impulses—also called the five positive emotions appear to have physical locations in the body," he explained, "but, actually they are points of contact between the physical body and the finer bodies. Unlike so much of what we human beings perceive, these impulses are not dualistic. They don't have a good aspect and a bad aspect. They are simply stronger or weaker and can be strengthened through meditative exercise."

In explaining their meaning, Bennett told us, "We often spoil them by interpreting them in the wrong way. We *Wish* to have something, *Hope* for results, *Believe* in creeds or people, use *Will* to do our own bidding, and *Love* with an agenda."

The only way I could begin to grasp his uncommon explanation was to think of them as qualities that stood alone rather than as actions with an object.

"We must look at these real emotions in a different way," Bennett said, "understanding that they are inside ourselves. They are our Oneness with Spirit—totally unlike our painful looking to something outside ourselves."

The first time during the course when Bennett arranged to meet each student privately was after we had practiced for several weeks meditative exercises attending to these sacred impulses. He asked us to observe our experience, intimating that we would be able to sense differences in strength among them. When I met with him, he asked, "What did you find to be your weak emotion?"

Unable to sense any differences, I just said what I thought. "I've often felt so hopeless, yet I've always believed that something existed inside or beyond ourselves."

Aware I did not have a clue, he didn't engage me in discussion, instead, he simply informed me, "It is *Belief* that you lack."

Unable to comprehend the difference between Hope and Belief, my thoughts scrambled to keep up with the rest of his words. All I remembered afterward was his imperative to watch, study, come to understand.

Now, these 30-odd years later, something in my relationship with you, Berry, awakened a need to discern between *Hope* and *Belief*. Our time together was calling up a slowly dawning comprehension. What was the purpose of the stories I had felt driven to go over? Except for the background about my parents, each one pointed to something beyond death—sensed, communicated from outside my ordinary physical existence and the consensual precepts of the culture.

Berry asked, How many times had I told you that our fears are the result of lacking *Belief*?

I tried to answer my own question, What is *Belief* without believing IN something? Contact with the immortal part of us? Life-beyond-life? Soul? That-which-is-greater-than-the-physical-world? I finally saw that, indeed, I'd always had *Hope*. I'd always kept searching, even in times of repeated despair. It was *Belief* that had been lacking. Didn't I always think those magical events were real only for other people—saints or chosen ones? My experiences were a mere glimmer, a pale shadow, not up to muster.

What it came down to was a matter of choice. To have no *Belief* was my pretense at sophistication. What it meant in daily life was despair, giving up. It was depressing. In those moments where *Belief* came uninvited—moments of grace—there was acceptance, trust, guidance, creativity, connection, surprises, even fun! Why would we be given such pleasures if they didn't have a sacred function?

During the time Berry and I were sorting through these thoughts, I was invited to join a discussion group with old friends. They had just read *Mutant Message Down Under*. I'd read it years before when it was first published and, now, I read it again. It is the story, the truth of which is still disputed, of a surprise walka-bout given as a gift to a woman who worked in Australia with aboriginal youth in the city. The aborigines told the author that fear was an emotion of the animal kingdom where it plays an important role in survival. "But if humans know about Divine Oneness and understand that the universe is not a haphazard event but an unfolding plan, they cannot be fearful. You either have faith or fear, not both."

The Hound of Heaven

Don't you wish there were a knob on the TV
to turn up the intelligence?
There's one marked "Brightness," but it doesn't work.
- GALLAGHER

The Berry thought asked me, Remember the poetry assignment I had given you?

I recalled a day when Berry had said once again, "I have an assignment for you. Would you go to the library and see if you can get a copy of Francis Thompson's poem, *The Hound of Heaven?*"

Oh, yes, I remember. I found it that afternoon in a worn old volume of English poetry. I had tried reading it before bringing it to you, but the obscure nineteenth century language put me off and I didn't get very far. You had been so pleased I'd found it.

"Read it to me," you said. Then you lay back and closed your intense dark eyes. I could sense you taking the poem in—as if you were eating fresh hummus. My task of reading it got me through it that time, but when you asked how I liked it I had to confess I barely had a clue to it's meaning.

"We'll go over it, line by line, if need be, and then it'll become clear to you," you had said serenely. "Go ahead, read it again." I read the first stanza.

> I fled Him, down the nights and down the days;
> I fled Him down the arches of the years;
> I fled Him, down the labyrinthine ways
>   Of my own mind, and in the mist of tears
> I hid from Him, and under running laughter.
>   Up vistaed hopes I sped;
>   And shot, precipitated,
> Adown Titanic glooms of chasmed fears,
> From those strong Feet that followed, followed after.
>   But with unhurrying chase,
>   And unperturbed pace,
>   Deliberate speed, majestic instancy,
>   They beat—and a Voice beat
>   More instant than the Feet—
> "All things betray thee, who betrayest Me...."

At that point you questioned me, "What is your sense of this part?"

"The 'H' in Him is capitalized so I have the feeling the poet is fleeing God—who appeared in many different circumstances," I had answered uncertainly.

You nodded and had me continue. At intervals you spoke

about the feeling and the imagery, sometimes clarifying the meaning of a line just by repeating what I had read, but using your own rhythm and flow. We spent the whole visit going over it. When you spoke, I understood, your appreciation seeming to enter me. I photocopied the poem and put it into my journal, never making any notes about the lesson.

A year after your death, I am reading the poem again. In detail it seems almost as unclear as it had originally except now it's imbued with you and the depth of its message.

I sense from its five pages of imagery how we wander or flee through life seeking love and comfort in so many ways, yet, repeatedly causing our own misery by denying Spirit which hounds us in its never-ending attempt to provide that which we seek.

> "....Ah, fondest, blindest, weakest,
> I am He Whom thou seekest!
> Thou dravest* love from thee, who dravest Me."

*drave=drive

Berry had not just been randomly selecting classics for me to read. The works she had chosen spoke directly to concerns I was grappling with, issues awakened by the experiences I had been driven to write about. Driven. Hounded to share with Berry, who would help me take them in.

The Last Revision

Thanks to impermanence, everything is possible.
- THICH NHAT HANH

When I finished the second draft, Berry urged me again, Take a break from the manuscript. It's the perfect time. You still don't appreciate how much perspective you'll gain, do you? Then, she added a carrot, Someone could be reading it while you rest.

It was December. There was plenty to be preoccupied with over the holidays. What I wanted now was feedback on the structure of the book although I'd already cut more than 100 pages and had interwoven Berry's and my relationship with the stories we worked on.

I found Ina, a creative writing instructor at the local college. We discussed what I wanted. I trusted her clarity. Nevertheless, I knew that whatever she said would launch me into more unknown territory where only hard work would bring back order.

After she read the manuscript, we met in her sparsely furnished office. First thing she said was, "Tell me again what you intended the book to be about."

"It's about belief and reality," I said. "It's about this person, me, who has numerous mysterious events happen throughout her life. Although they feel special, I can't quite believe their reality, at least not enough to actually integrate them into my life." I continued, "And all of that hangs on the framework of my relationship with Berry. Something about Berry's complete acceptance makes me go over these events and come into a different relationship with them."

"Yes," said Ina, "I asked because in its present form there are two equally weighted themes throughout the book. The relationship with Berry and the philosophical angle about reality. But what you just said is the key. Any philosophy of interest hangs on the armature of your relationship with Berry. An ideology is not what the book is about. Readers aren't going to be hooked by philosophical discourse. It is the relationship that they'll care about. It's

259

a love story!"

A love story! Berry and I repeated in unison.

Then Ina described in her own way what I had experienced. "Berry parented you in a manner you hadn't been parented and you appreciated her in a way that couldn't happen in her other relationships, possibly because of the alcoholism. She may have parented you to a degree she hadn't been able to parent her own children. Berry's mentoring was healing, bringing about an acceptance of your own mystical reality."

I said, "The circumstances of our lives created this secure environment where we both played out an unforseen scenario..." I began to tear up but squelched it.

When Ina began talking again, I started taking notes. She stopped speaking and I looked up at her, noting her dark eyes and hair starkly contrasting with her almost luminous skin. She said stiffly, "Before you write, I want to talk. Then I'll go over the points that are important so you won't lose them. Just give me your full attention now."

I bristled at the dogmatic tone, but understood what she was suggesting.

Softening her inflection, she said, "I was confused because you told me it was a memoir, yet most of it is written in the third person."

"I'd gone back and forth about that," I said, "but now, I realize by having written it in the third person, I still wasn't owning the events I had been rejecting all my life. The struggle about which person to use was another clue to what writing the book was revealing. I'm sure now, it's going to be in the first person."

"If it is," Ina explained, "you can get away with having so much of your point of view in it. But in the third person, it needs to be more balanced, showing as much about Berry as about you."

When Ina had gone over her concerns, she announced, "Okay, it's time for the summary." I picked up my pen and dutifully held it poised against the sheet I had been writing on.

"...on a fresh piece of paper," she said.

I resisted.

"On a fresh piece of paper," she repeated.

Hackles rising, I didn't actually say the words to myself but just felt, This is my journal I'm writing in, for godsake! I've been keeping it for forty-five years. I'll write on whatever damned page I want. I hunkered down waiting for Ina to continue, which, upon seeing my resolve, she did.

Berry was clucking at me the whole time, but I couldn't stop my reaction.

I'm sure something good could come of that characteristic, she said, thoughtfully giving me the benefit of the doubt...or was that a euphemistic distortion disguised as praise? She laughed, pleased with herself.

Ina made her points and concluded in summary, "Through Berry's memoirs, she bequeathes her life experiences to you which you accept unconditionally. Ultimately, you both feel acknowledgement from each other which neither of you previously received."

Elik

The most beautiful thing we can experience is the mysterious.
It is the source of all true art and science.
- ALBERT EINSTEIN

Completing the manuscript seemed like it was involving more and more people, everyone around me uncovering some piece of the story. Every topic of discussion, every observation seemed relevant. My focused eighteen month isolation was dissolving.

Across the table sat Elik. How long had I known her? More than twenty years. Long enough for her dark hair to turn gray and mine to turn gray, red, blondish, and gray, again. She complimented me on my mismatched earrings. We share a penchant for asymmetry. I'd just begun the third draft and was in a funk.

"After not looking at it for a month and a half," I lamented, "now that I've read it afresh and taken in Ina's comments, I can see the lack of direction and rhythm. It's choppy and off-balance with long philosophical discourses."

Elik giggled. "She's here," Elik said, looking to the empty space in the booth at my right side. "She wants to help you."

It took me a minute to realize who she was talking about.

"Berry?"

Elik nodded. Elik sees metaphors or that's the closest description we've come up with. Sometimes they're spirits. They're very helpful. Except when she let the wrong people know about them. But that was when she was still trying to please those closest and most critical of her, allowing them to determine how she should perceive reality.

Elik closed her eyes and said. "Berry is showing me a picture. You're sitting on a hill, way up, overlooking a beautiful valley. There's also a tree up there, nearby. The trunk is twisted. So are the branches—twisted and pointy. Dead. It's dead. It's the past. It doesn't have anything to do with you. You're there and it's there, but you're separate. Now, it's spring and everything is green, beautiful. The tree is from when things were hard, dry, convoluted."

I said, looking over at non-physical Berry, "Do you mean, when life felt so limited, when it took so much effort...?"

"She means," Elik said, lifting her chin toward Berry, "if I may speak for you?" and then looked furtively around the restaurant laughing again. "I'm just looking to see if anyone is watching us talk with a person who isn't here."

I laughed, too, then shrugged.

Elik closed her eyes again. "She's showing us how the stream is meandering down the mountain, saying 'Just let the story flow.'" Elik gestures with her hand, waving it back and forth to show switchbacks. I write the word 'serpentine' and show it to her.

"Did you write that first?"

"No. The image just reminded me of a word Berry used with

me all the time. It referred to a number of things—how we could hold contradictory feelings in our awareness, saying them, just being honest, showing our layered experience, but often making people angry because the words went against the norm. To us they were just different viewpoints that were apparent."

Then Berry reminded me of another concept she introduced me to, relating to flow. I described it to Elik. "In writing, Berry would infer something—she called it being elliptical—speaking around something to let people figure out the possibilities for themselves. Berry encouraged me, saying, 'Accept your perceptions and express them, but not necessarily directly. You're afraid of your thoughts because you know there will be reactions. But when you hide your thoughts completely, your caution makes people suspicious. They sense something is being covered up. It works against you.'"

Following Ina's idea of clarifying the theme and Berry's idea of flow, it was easy to cut another 113 pages and change transitions throughout the manuscript. Then, as I finished rereading new material for the last section, Berry said sympathetically, I know most of it is new but...it's got to go.

How was this going to play itself out? I asked myself as I reached over to the bookshelf and pulled down Tara's gift from a few years before, *Walking on Alligators: Daily meditations for writers*. As I opened it heedlessly, I mused, I haven't looked at this for a long time. My eyes focused on the quote at the top of the page. It was from Voltaire. "The secret of being tiresome is to tell everything."

The Personal Totem

And now here is my secret, a very simple secret:
It is only with the heart that one can see rightly;
what is essential is invisible to the eye.

- ANTOINE DE SAINT-EXUPÉRY FROM THE LITTLE PRINCE

Amidst the new flurry of activity in my life, I embarked on examining my old diaries. They became noticeably more interesting in the 90s when the newly developing optimism included notes from conferences, inner exercises, coincidences.

I came upon an exercise I'd done and written up a couple of years before meeting Berry. *The Personal Totem Pole,* a book by Stephen Gallegos suggests meditatively identifying an animal at each of the seven chakras—the energy vortices associated with the body as described in Hindu philosophy.

During my experiment with the exercise, animals appeared which although different from the ones the author experienced, nevertheless, seemed appropriate to the function of the chakra and my experiences. The next step was to converse with them to bring new awareness.

Following-up on the exercise, now over two years later, Gallegos suggested checking in with each chakra individually to see if the animal had changed. "If it has, ask if it is important for you to know what was happening in your life that corresponds with the change."

When I got to the third chakra, my blousy yellow butterfly whom I had begun to think of as Berry was there, delicate and colorful.

She said, "I want you to know I'm retiring. Do think of me as Berry—retiring to the spirit world." And then she made the announcement, "Bat will be taking my place."

"Bat?!" I actually burst into tears, complaining, "Bats are scary! They fly so erratically."

My tears set off a commotion, all the chakra animals talking at once, trying to calm me.

"Bat is a warm-blooded mammal."

"...with more substance."

"He flies irregularly but not from lacking control."

"...sensitive self-control, radar."

"...catching insects on the move in the dark!"

"...directs himself in the night, moving easily through the unseen world."

I echoed the words slowly, "...*moving easily through the unseen world*," suddenly becoming placid, my tears drying up as I breathed in deeply an unexpected sense of promise.

After rereading the entire manuscript once again, I put it down to make myself a cup of tea. Was that the ending? I wasn't sure.

I returned to my desk, lost in thought, and mindlessly opened *Walking On Alligators* as I pulled it down from the shelf again. Awakening to its presence in my hands, I looked down and read, "We work in the dark. We really don't know what the final outcome of our writing will be. We don't know what the book...will look like when printed. We don't know what effect it will have on readers. We don't even know what effect it will have on us when we reread it....We all go forward by faith in the task."

Acknowledgments

Prayer is not an old woman's idle amusement.
Properly understood and applied,
it is the most potent instrument of action.
- MAHATMA GANDHI

I am grateful for all the help and pleasure that has come my way while this book was being born. Thanks to Tara Bell, my personal cheerleader and book midwife who was so often available when needed. To the memory of her sister-in-law Janice who seemed to accompany us during much of the journey. To my loving husband, Bruce Appelgren, who seems confident that I can write about anything, dear brother Jerry Koppel and his devoted wife Linda who uplift me with their good will, to my conscientious parents Shirley and Emanuel Koppel who made more things possible than they could have imagined, to grandparents George and Anna (Halperin) Koppel and Israel and Rose (Goldstein) Markin who courageously left all that they knew in the Old World to help create the New World, mysterious ancestor, Israel's grandmother, Laughing Woman, to our three sympathetic nieces, Laura, Trish, and Lynn, and their loving mother Geraldine.

There are people and their organizations who inspired experiences with the otherworld which helped me break through the wall of rationalism that has bogged me down—John G.Bennett and the International Society for Continuous Education at Sherborne House, John Broomfield, Edgar Cayce and the Association for Research and Enlightenment, David Davidson, Elik, Gerald Epstein, M.D., Eligio Stephen Gallegos, Elmer Green and the International Society for the Study of Subtle Energies and Energy Medicine, David Hawkins, Carl G. Jung, Eka Kapiotis, Neil Lamper and Gestalt Psychology, The Monroe Institute, Bellruth Naparstek, Rebekah Rice Riley, Dana Robinson, Martin Rossman, the School of the Art Institute of Chicago, Linda Schiller-Hannah, June Singer, and Tom who became Alois.

Visitors from the Otherworld have often surprised me with

information and humor, a gift that directs us like a beacon—dauntless crocodile who started it all, aborigines of Australia, steadfast bat, blousy yellow butterfly, the chakra council, Granny D., and oryx.

There are many who just seem to exude a confidence in me that provided supportive energy for which I am grateful—Hester Balsam, Jim Barbour and the gods of the circumstances, Geoff Byrd, Georgia DuBose, Grace Earl, Ruthie and Ian Fingerman, Barbara Goree, Crystal Hawk, Jack Houck, Emanuel Jacobson, Don Kingman, Robert Ochs, Veronica Phillips, R.W. Roberts, Elva and Edward Schneidman, Joel Shepperd, M.D., Betsy and Peter Shor, Roy Silverstein, Harry and Vera Sirota, Alexandra and Dan Sperling, Edith Wallace, M.D., Philip B. Welch, Dr. Ralph Yochim,

Bruce Appelgren, Tara Bell, Alice L. McElhinney, Ilona Popper, and Marge Thelan read through the entire manuscript at different stages and gave me invaluable advice. Marge wishes me "good writing' almost daily. Judith Stevens and Joyce Lerner contributed copyediting along with renewed friendship. I am, however, responsible for any remaining errors.

The Berryville Writers' Read and Critique Group (Empress Kathleen McDaniel, Tara Bell, Millie Curtis, Ringo McDaniel, Lee Person, Marge Thelen, Audria Carroll, and Dick Bell) listened to parts of the manuscript for weeks on end, sharing experience, giving supportive feedback, and generally being optimistic. We also shared much laughter, that most nourishing food. And what an interesting variety of manuscripts they have! I always looked forward to our 'story hours'.

Martha Koelling was my second grade teacher who valued her students and made us think words were fun. Although I never met them, writers Susan Shaunessy (*Walking on Alligators: A Book Of Meditations For Writers*) and Susan Page (*The Shortest Distance Between You And A Published Book*), through their books, accompanied and inspired the process of writing this one.

I mention Bill and Miriam Gough for their kindness and great work in examining the 'white crows' in life, Stef for her most valuable lessons about compassion and Steve for his generosity,

Curmudgeon.com for making available so much wisdom, the Healing Arts Council of the Shenandoah Valley (Rose Atwood, Michael Rohrbacher, Janet Romero, Joanne Royaltey, Carol Weare, Clair and Jack Bellingham, Julianna Fehr, Andrea Frye, Cathleen McCoy, and Tom Schulz) for all the laughs and meaningful projects, the Shenandoah Alliance for the Healing Arts for introducing me to people whose Belief and healing energies touch so many others, Christine Ziemnik my distant apartment mate who brought an abundance of playful schemes into my life, Joe Z. and his family of origin for graciously inviting me to participate during a significant time of their lives, and Berry Morgan's daughter who so generously shared her mother with me.

Where does one draw the line with such a list? If I have not recognized the immediate influence of someone on the production of this book, forgive me and pray for my illumination. Thanks also to friends and acquaintances who enrich life daily and with whom I travel on the planetary sojourn.

From BJ Appelgren's next book...

Freshly Laundered And Hanging Out To Dry [©]

The best time to plant a tree was twenty years ago.
The second best time is now.
-CHINESE PROVERB

Preface

I didn't think of myself as a hippie, but travelling through Europe, that's what people called me. Who else would travel without an itinerary, carrying only a backpack for months of travel, not knowing when she was going home? Who else but a young American had the wealth and freedom to do that?

I tried to understand what defined me and my peers. When I had been growing up in Chicago, my schoolmates were mostly first- and second-generation Americans. The neighborhood was Swedish Lutheran, Irish Catholic, and Russian Jewish. Had our families still been living in the Old World, we never would have met. I think this exposure was significant, allowing us to know each other beyond the national origins and religious customs to which we were still connected.

By the 1960s, we were the first generation to have had an unprecedented seventeen years of schooling. The American economy was completely recovered from the Great Depression which had delineated our parents' young adulthood. Not only were we educated, we had a choice of jobs open to us.

About the time I got out of college, however, I remember a feeling of dissatisfaction hovering in the air. Discrimination against blacks and gender disparities conflicted with the democratic ideals we'd studied about in school. When I travelled I learned that, indeed, I was rich compared to people living in the countries visited. At the same time, by more traditional American standards, I was practically a vagabond.

I was looking for something, not really knowing what. I'd explored social activism and learned that the radical organizations created to bypass greed and power hunger, exhibited the very same traits as the so-called establishment. So I continued searching elsewhere.

I don't know what the figures were but when I began to travel around Europe and through the Near East, I discovered droves of other Americans doing the same thing, even into the Far East. We didn't travel like older American tourists but more like European ones, riding third class, hitchhiking, camping, staying at hostels, or wherever we were invited for free.

We began exploring spiritual avenues, too, perhaps not intentionally at first—just coming upon meditation and Eastern religions accidently, then being touched by those experiences in ways we hadn't known before.

It wasn't until I'd returned to Chicago, after seven months of wandering, that a series of coincidences led me to a life-defining experience—a ten-month practicum in spiritual transformation. I was so driven and hungry for its promise, I couldn't have been kept away.

Yet once there, I discovered it wasn't pleasant or easy. Many times during the course I stayed only because I'd made a commitment, knowing there was an end in sight. I'm glad I stayed because, over the last thirty-two years, it has continued to be a living force in my life.

To contact the author for readings, writing workshops, and pre-sentations, go to the website http://www.TransparentFeather.com